Beauty Recipes

Ultimate Cookbook and Beginner's Guide to Eating for Youthful Skin and Energy

Table Of Contents

I want to thank you and congratulate you for getting started with the book, *"Beauty Recipes – Ultimate Cookbook and Beginner's Guide to Eating for Youthful Skin and Energy"*.

Chapter 1: How Processed Food Puts Strain on Your Body, Causes Aging, and Drains Energy

Your diet can significantly affect the way you look. If you want your skin to be smooth, soft, and supple, you have to avoid consuming processed foods, such as processed meat, pasteurized dairy products, and refined grains. These products contain high levels of phosphates, which are used as flavor enhancers and preservatives. They accelerate the signs of aging as well as put you at risk of developing other complications, such as cardiovascular calcification and kidney disease. In addition, they can lead to skin and muscle atrophy.

Researchers state that high levels of phosphate can also be found in sodas. They are used to react with sodium bicarbonate and produce fizz (or carbon dioxide). Hence, you should also limit or avoid the consumption of such beverages. As mentioned earlier, high levels of phosphate can accelerate aging and contribute to complications associated with age. If you want to live a long life and enjoy the benefits of good health, you should keep the phosphates in your diet balanced.

Another reason why you should stop drinking sodas is because of the phosphorus they contain. This mineral is added to sodas, in the form of phosphoric acid, to give these beverages their tangy taste, as well as act as preservatives. Although phosphorus is vital in keeping your teeth and bones healthy, it can also be damaging if not taken in the right amounts. According to research, phosphorus can influence aging, which is why it is crucial to keep it balanced.

What's more, drinking sodas can cause loss of bone mass, brittle bones, muscle weakness, paralysis, pancreatic cancer, type-2 diabetes, obesity, mineral imbalance, and addiction to caffeine. In fact, drinking just a couple of cans of soda a week can already increase your risk of developing these diseases. If you think that drinking sodas can give you an energy boost, you are wrong. They can actually deprive you of the energy you need to complete your tasks.

Refined grains are not really good for you because they already have their nutritional values stripped off. They have the same effect on your body as sugar. Sugar actually provokes chronic inflammation and makes you age more quickly. Hence, you should avoid brown sugar, table sugar, raw sugar, sorghum syrup, maple syrup, rice syrup, corn sweetener, molasses, dextrose, liquid cane sugar, glucose, fructose, concentrated fruit juices, and barley malt.

Anyway, refined grains also have additional ingredients that make them worse for your health. These ingredients include sugar, artificial ingredients, and excess salt. So, when you go to the grocery store, see to it that you do not pick up white flour, white rice, white bread, pasta, noodles, baked goods, and biscuits. White flour (or refined flour) can clog up your bowels, cause obesity or weight gain, and apply pressure on your digestive system. It is nothing but empty calories – and of course, it can accelerate aging.

Baked goods also contain acrylamides, carcinogenic chemicals that accelerate aging and increase the risk of cancer. Processed foods also typically contain trans fats or hydrogenated fats. These are artificial fats that accelerate aging, as well as promote inflammation, obesity, high cholesterol, and insulin resistance. You can also get breakouts and acne from eating fried and processed foods.

Chapter 2: Should You Be Confused with the Different Diets Available?

At present, there are a lot of diets available. You can find diets that claim to help people lose weight, build muscle, or have clearer skin. If you want your skin to be smoother and more radiant, you can try out diets that promise such effects. Nonetheless, see to it that the diet you follow is legitimate, safe, and effective. Sadly, a huge percentage of the diets available are bogus and ineffective.

There are plenty of diets that are not helpful at all. Most of these are actually just fad diets. Such diets are typically restricting. They tell dieters to limit their food intake or not eat at all. Numerous people believe that these diets can help them achieve their target output. In reality though, these diets are unhealthy and ineffective. Instead of helping you achieve your goal, you will actually end up feeling worse.

On the bright side, there are also lots of legit, safe, and effective diets. You can research about them, so you can acquire more information. Several magazines and journals contain vital information about these diets. Furthermore, you can use the Internet for your research. You can find blogs, articles, and review sites that tell you more about the different types of diets available today.

Then again, you have to do a lot of research before you try following a particular diet. Your health is not something that you should risk. Therefore, it is crucial to gather all the necessary information regarding the diet that you want to pursue. If you want to have clearer and younger-looking skin, it is only proper that you look for a diet that is healthy and approved by the Food and Drug Administration.

In addition, make sure that you read reviews about these diets. You may get confused with the vast availability of these diets. The information they provide might also be confusing. If you want a diet that can help you have clearer and more beautiful skin, you should consider diets that claim to help dieters get rid of acne, rashes, age spots, wrinkles, fine lines, crow's feet, and other skin blemishes.

Keep in mind that these diets should include tips on eating the right kinds of food and using the right kinds of skin products. If you read anything that tells you to stop eating for a few days or solely depend on a particular supplement or drug, you should stay away from it. A good diet will never tell you to compromise your health and safety. You should use your common sense when searching for diets.

Moreover, you can ask your doctor for help. Professional advice might be necessary if you are really having a hard time looking for the right diet. Your dermatologist can also recommend a diet that is suitable for you. Such a skincare expert can even create a custom diet depending on your physical condition. A custom diet may be ideal (and even necessary) if you have any existing skin condition or if you are taking some kind of prescription medication.

Chapter 3: Natural Foods that are Sugar-, Gluten-, Grain-, and Dairy-Free Work Best for Your Body

From the previous chapters, you have learned why unprocessed foods are bad for your skin. So, if you really want to have clearer and healthier skin, you should have a good diet. Keep in mind that it is not enough to use skin care products alone. No matter how much anti-aging cream or lotion you apply, your skin's condition would still not improve if you do not take care of your health.

You should take care of your body not just externally, but also internally. In fact, it is more important to take care of your body internally. Even if you do not buy expensive skin care products, you will still have great skin if you follow of a healthy diet. Your skin will glow with health if you drink lots of water and eat fruits, vegetables, and lean proteins.

When it comes to food, lots of people favor taste over nutritive value. They eat tasty yet unhealthy food, which is why they become overweight, sickly, and weak. Good thing is, there are sugar-, gluten-, dairy-, and grain-free diets that can help improve your skin, mood, and energy levels. These diets can also help you lose and maintain your ideal weight.

So, why are gluten, dairy, grains, and sugar bad for your skin? Well, these food products can cause inflammation, and inflammation can result in psoriasis, dermatitis, eczema, acne, and other skin problems. Eating these foods can make your skin irritated and reddish. Similarly, these foods can make you lose energy, become moody and irritable, and increase your risks of suffering from various diseases.

On the other hand, natural foods that are processed sugar-, gluten-, dairy-, and grain-free are great for your overall health. When you are on these diets, you should avoid foods that contain barley, wheat, rye, additives, refined sugar, and milk. The hormones contained in milk can increase your androgen levels and trigger oil production, causing your pores to clog.

Sugar can cause your body to produce an insulin-like growth factor and trigger inflammation. The glucose in sugar can also stress out your skin, as well as trigger enzymes (such as elastin and collagen) that can break down your skin tissues. This will cause your skin to age faster. So, if you want to stay young-looking, energetic, and healthy, you should choose natural foods.

Vegetables are highly recommended since they are full of antioxidants, which slow down the aging process and fight against free radicals. Kale, spinach, and other green, leafy vegetables contain the highest amounts of antioxidants, including zeaxanthin and lutin. These antioxidants have been found to be effective in protecting the skin against the harmful ultraviolet rays of the sun.

Aside from antioxidants, vegetables are also full of vitamins and minerals, such as vitamins A, C, E, and K. They are ideal for the immune system, and they can help prevent high blood pressure and cardiovascular disease. Orange-red vegetables are excellent too. These vegetables contain large amounts of beta-carotene, which are converted into vitamin A by your body. This vitamin can prevent premature aging and cell damage.

Alkaline-forming foods, such as almonds, lemons, pears, parsley, and kale are also highly recommended if you want to have younger-looking skin. You can also consume walnuts and wild Alaskan salmon. These foods contain omega-3 fatty acids and can keep your skin hydrated. Keep in mind that keeping your skin hydrated is a must if you do not want to have wrinkles.

Do not forget to eat tomatoes, as they are rich in lycopene. This phytochemical helps get rid of free radicals that cause the skin to age. It protects your skin against the damaging ultraviolet rays of the sun. If you want to prevent sunburn, you should eat half a cup of cooked tomatoes on a daily basis, as well as apply sunscreen protection. It is important to take note that tomatoes release lycopene when they are cooked.

Nuts are great anti-aging foods too. They contain protein and unsaturated fats. They contain omega-3 fatty acids, as well as potassium and vitamin E. However, nuts are quite heavy on the calories, which is why it is ideal to eat only a handful. If you are watching your weight, see to it that you do not consume too many nuts. Nonetheless, nuts can keep you satiated, so you do not have to eat a lot throughout the day.

As you know, vitamin E is an antioxidant that can maintain the youthful glow of your skin. It can also help you maintain good eyesight. Nuts also contain selenium, zinc, and omega-3 fatty acids, all of which have the same positive effect on the skin. Particularly, zinc maintains collagen, so the micronutrient helps your skin stay firm, smooth, and supple. Zinc, along with biotin and vitamin B6, also keeps your hair shiny.

If you'd have a glass of red wine every day, you will also have better-looking skin because red wine has nutrients and antioxidants that are good for your body. It actually contains resveratrol, an antioxidant that slows down the aging process as well as prevents blood clots, reduce inflammation, lower bad cholesterol, and prevent cancer. The alcohol content of red wine can also increase your levels of good cholesterol.

You should also eat avocados, as these fruits are well-known for their anti-aging properties. They contain potassium, vitamin E, antioxidants, and monounsaturated fats. The vitamins and minerals that avocados contain can lower blood pressure, reduce cholesterol, and improve the condition of the skin. Also, avocados contain vitamin B or folic acid, which is useful in preventing osteoporosis.

Citrus fruits are good eats, as well. They can help your body produce collagen. Collagen is actually the protein that composes your skin's basic structure and, as mentioned earlier, it is necessary in keeping your skin firm, smooth, and supple. Without sufficient collagen, your skin will be saggy. Hence, you need the vitamin C that citrus fruits contain to tighten your skin.

Other natural foods that can stimulate collagen production are sweet potatoes. These foods are rich in vitamin C, which efficiently boost collagen production and eliminate wrinkles. According to a study published in the American Journal of Clinical Nutrition, individuals who ate half a sweet potato every day for three years were able to decrease their wrinkles by 11 percent.

Mangoes, apricots, and papayas are rich in carotenoids, which are also good for your skin. If you eat these fruits, your skin will have a rosy glow. So, if your skin looks dull, stop lathering on some beauty product and have a serving of these fruits instead. You can also have mussels because they are rich in iron. If your body does not have sufficient iron, your skin will be pasty and pale.

Natural foods that are rich in antioxidants and phytonutrients are highly recommended to those who want to age gracefully and improve their overall health. Phytonutrients are organic components found in plants. They are essential in the prevention of various diseases and premature aging. Antioxidants are molecules that prevent or slow down molecule oxidation. This also allows them to fight free radicals.

You can get antioxidants and phytonutrients from berries, including raspberries, blackberries, cherries, blueberries, and strawberries. You should focus on eating berries and vegetables that are rich in fiber. Again, you should limit or avoid consuming processed foods. If you have a sweet tooth, you can get "natural sugar" from fruits, such as bananas and apples.

It is crucial to keep the levels of insulin in your body steady, so you can slow down your aging process. You should consume low-glycemic index foods that do not increase or spike insulin. Some of the natural foods that are rich in antioxidants and have low-glycemic indexes are asparagus, bell pepper, Brussels sprouts, chili pepper, garlic, onion, ginger, fish, fish oil, olive oil, and parsley.

As mentioned earlier, your skin also needs vitamin E in order to maintain its radiance and health. Without sufficient amounts of this vitamin, your skin will be dull, dry, and flaky. While there are lots of manufacturers that claim to produce vitamin E supplements, it is still much better to obtain vitamin E from natural sources. Synthetic forms of vitamins may be dangerous.

If you are over forty, chances are you are lacking in omega-3 (and also in EPA and DHA fatty acids). Unfortunately, people tend to be more deficient in these nutrients as they grow older. So, if you want to avoid serious diseases, premature aging, and loss of energy, see to it that your body gets sufficient nutrients. Then again, make sure that you stay away from omega-3 supplements that contain low-grade ingredients.

Likewise, you should be careful when choosing protein sources. When you reach the age of forty, your muscle mass starts to decline. As you grow even older, your muscle mass declines further. Hence, you should make sure that you get enough protein. Choose meats that came from animals that were given diets that don't involve herbicides and pesticides. You can also have organic legumes as your source of protein.

Beauty Recipes

Breakfast Recipes

Chicken Breakfast Patties
Crunchy Grain-Free Granola
Carrot Cake Pancakes
Bacon and Sweet Potato Hash
Apple and Pulled Pork Hashcakes
Ham, Egg & Veggie Breakfast Burrito
Breakfast Pizza
Turkey Bacon Club Salad
Cobb Salad
Crab Cakes
No-Oats Oatmeal
Acorn Squash 'N Eggs
Beef and Plantain Stir-Fry
Tuna Spread
Egg In A Hole
Apple Nut Bake
Bacon & Fruit Scramble
Salmon & Veggie Breakfast Salad
Cowboy Breakfast Skillet
Creole Frittata
Coconut and Banana Pancakes
Pumpkin & Bacon Pancakes
Tapioca Blueberry Crepes

Cashew Belgian Waffles
Apple Upside Down Cakes

Chicken Breakfast Patties

Prep Time: 5 minutes

Cook Time: 10 minutes

Servings: 2

INGREDIENTS

8 oz chicken

1 egg

1/4 cup coconut flour

1/2 sweet onion

1 tablespoon apple cider vinegar

1 teaspoon ground black pepper

1 teaspoon sea salt

1 teaspoon paprika

1 teaspoon ground sage

1 teaspoon dried thyme

1 teaspoon fennel seed (optional)

1/2 teaspoon nutmeg (optional)

1 tablespoon water

Coconut oil (for cooking)

INSTRUCTIONS

1. Heat medium skillet over medium heat and lightly coat with coconut oil.

2. Grind chicken meat and peeled 1/2 onion to medium grind in food processor, bullet blender, or meat grinder. Or grind onion alone and add to pre-ground chicken in medium bowl.

3. Add apple cider vinegar, spices and 1 tablespoon coconut flour to ground chicken and onion. Mix well until combined. Form into 2 large or 4 small patties and place on plate.

4. Beat egg with water and pour egg wash over patties. Gently flip patties to get them evenly covered with egg wash. Take coconut flour and sprinkle over both sides of egg washed patties. Pat coconut flour gently into patties.

5. Place coated patties into hot oiled skillet and cook about 3 - 4 minutes, until golden brown and crisp. Flip and cook another 3 - 4 minutes, or until done.

6. Remove cooked patties from pan and drain on paper towel. Serve hot.

Crunchy Grain-Free Granola

Prep Time: 5 minutes

Cook Time: 20 minutes

Servings: 4

INGREDIENTS

1 cup almond flour

1/4 cup ground chia seed (or flax seed meal)

1 tablespoon vanilla

1 teaspoon ground nutmeg

1 teaspoon ground cinnamon

1/2 cup raw agave nectar (or 1/2 cup raw honey + 1 tablespoon water)

1 cup flaked coconut

1 cup sliced almonds

1/2 cup dried figs

1/2 cup dried dates

1/2 cup pecans

1/2 cup pumpkin seeds

1/2 cup dried apricots

1/2 cup coconut oil, melted

INSTRUCTIONS

1. Preheat oven to 350 degrees F. Lightly coat cookie sheet with coconut oil.

2. Stem figs and pit dates. Chop figs, dates, pecans and apricots. Add to medium bowl, along with all other ingredients. Mix to combine, then spread evenly over sheet pan with spatula.

3. Bake in preheated oven for about 10 minutes. Then carefully remove and use spatula to turn over par-baked granola. Bake for additional 8 - 10 minutes. Check periodically to ensure nuts do not over-toast.

4. Remove from oven and let cool and firm. Serve cool.

Carrot Cake Pancakes

Prep Time: 5 minutes

Cook Time: 15 minutes

Servings: 2

INGREDIENTS

1 3/4 cups almond meal

2 eggs

3/4 cup almond milk

2 medium carrots

1/4 cup chopped walnuts

1/4 cup golden raisins (optional)

1 teaspoon baking powder

1 tablespoon ground cinnamon

1 teaspoon ground nutmeg

1 teaspoon ground ginger

1 teaspoon vanilla

1/4 teaspoon sea salt

Pinch of ground black pepper

INSTRUCTIONS

1. Heat large skillet on medium-high heat and lightly coat with oil.
2. Finely grate carrots and drain in paper towel, or roughly process in food processor or bullet blender.
3. In medium bowl whisk eggs, almond milk, vanilla, cinnamon, nutmeg, ginger and black pepper.

4. Add almond flour, salt and baking powder. Whisk until smooth. Stir in carrots, walnuts and raisins (optional).

5. Use ladle or dry measure cup to pour 1/3 cup of batter onto hot oiled skillet. Fit 2 or 3 pancakes comfortably, so they do not touch as they spread.

6. Cook until sides of pancakes are firm and batter bubbles up a bit. About 3 - 4 minutes.

7. Carefully flip pancakes with spatula and cook for additional minute, or until cooked through. Repeat with remaining batter. Re-oil pan if necessary. Pancakes will be slightly delicate, so flip and plate with care.

8. Serve warm. Sprinkle with cinnamon and drizzle with agave nectar, or topping of choice.

Bacon and Sweet Potato Hash

Prep Time: 10 minutes

Cook Time: 10 minutes

Servings: 2

INGREDIENTS

8 oz nitrate-free bacon (thick cut slices or whole slab)

1 medium sweet potato

1 small white onion

1 teaspoon ground cinnamon

1 teaspoon dried thyme

1 teaspoon rosemary

INSTRUCTIONS

1. Bring medium pot to boil with lightly salted water. Leave enough room in pot for sweet potato. Heat a large skillet over high heat.

2. Chop bacon into 1/2 inch pieces or cubes. Add to hot skillet and brown. Stir occasionally with wooden spoon.

3. Peel and dice sweet potato. Add to boiling water for about 4 minutes, until tender but not mushy.

4. While potatoes and bacon cook, peel and dice onion.

5. Once browned, add onion to bacon. Sauté about 1 minute, until onions are tender and a bit caramelized.

6. Drain sweet potatoes in colander and add to skillet. Sprinkle on cinnamon, thyme and rosemary. Sauté 1 - 2 minutes, until any

excess liquid is evaporated and everything is lightly caramelized and cooked through. Serve hot.

Apple and Pulled Pork Hashcakes

Prep Time: 5 minutes

Cook Time: 10 minutes

Servings: 2

INGREDIENTS

Hashcakes:

8 oz pre-cooked pulled pork

1 tart apple

1 small white onion

1/4 – 1/2 cup almond flour

1 egg

Pinch ground black pepper

Pinch paprika

Pinch sea salt

Quick Grill Sauce:

8 oz (1 can) organic tomato sauce

1 sweet apple

2 whole roasted red peppers (jarred)

2 tablespoons organic mustard (or mustard powder)

1 tablespoon raw honey (optional)

1 oz apple cider vinegar

Pinch ground black pepper

Pinch paprika

Pinch cayenne pepper

Water

1. Heat large skillet over medium-high heat and lightly coat with coconut oil. Heat small pot over medium heat.

2. Blend all **Quick Grill Sauce** ingredients in food processor or bullet blender. Only add as much water as needed to get mixture smooth. Add to small pot and reduce until thickened to BBQ sauce consistency.

3. Beat egg in medium bowl with black pepper, paprika and salt. Peel and core apple. Grate apple and onion and add to medium bowl.

4. Lightly shred pulled pork and add to bowl. Sprinkling in almond flour a little at a time and mix with hand or wooden spoon. Get pulled pork mixture to just hold together in patty form. Do not over-flour or over mix.

5. Form 2 large or 4 small patties and gently lay into hot oiled skillet. Cook about 2 - 3 minutes, until golden brown and crisp. Flip and cook another 2 - 3 minutes, or until heated through and browned.

6. Remove cooked patties from pan and drain on paper towel. Serve hot.

Ham, Egg & Veggie Breakfast Burrito

Prep Time: 10 minutes

Cook Time: 10 minutes

Servings: 2

INGREDIENTS

Tortillas:

2 tablespoons coconut flour

2 tablespoons almond flour

2 teaspoons ground flax seed

2 eggs

2 tablespoons melted coconut oil

1/4 teaspoon baking powder

1/4 - 1/2 cup water

Coconut oil (for cooking)

Filling:

6 oz natural pre-cooked ham

6 eggs

1 bell pepper

1/2 red onion

1 avocado

4 oz organic salsa

Pinch sea salt

Pinch ground black pepper

INSTRUCTIONS

1. Heat large pan over medium-high heat and coat with 2 tablespoons of coconut oil. Heat second skillet over medium heat and lightly coat with coconut oil.

2. For *Tortillas*, blend coconut flour, almond flour, flax meal and baking powder in medium bowl. In separate bowl, whisk together 2 eggs, 2 tablespoons coconut oil and 1/4 cup water.

3. Slowly whisk dry blend into wet mixture. Whisk as you pour to avoid clumps. Continue to whisk and slowly add just enough water to make thin but hearty batter.

4. Once coconut oil is hot, use ladle or dry measure cup to pour half of batter into large pan. Tilt pan in circular motion as you pour so batter spreads thinly. Cook batter for about 2 minutes or until tortilla is slightly golden and firm.

5. While *Tortillas* cook, seed and stem pepper and peel onion. Chop ham, pepper and onion. Add to second skillet and sauté for about 2 minutes.

6. Flip tortilla and cook for 2 more minutes. Remove when toasted and cooked through. Place on paper towel or parchment. Add remaining batter to large pan, repeating tilting process to create thin tortilla.

7. While second tortilla cooks , beat 6 eggs in medium bowl and pour over veggies and ham. Salt and pepper to taste. Scramble until desired firmness.

8. Fill both tortillas down center each with half of ham scramble. Slice avocado in half, pit, then scoop out flesh onto each burrito.

9. Roll up tortillas and plate fold-side down. Dollop with your favorite salsa. Serve warm.

Breakfast Pizza

Prep Time: 10 minutes

Cook Time: 15 minutes

Servings: 2

INGREDIENTS

Crust:

1 1/2 cup almond flour

1/4 cup tablespoons coconut flour

2 eggs

1 tablespoon melted coconut oil

Coconut oil (for cooking)

Topping:

4 eggs

4 oz pre-cooked natural sausage

1/2 small red onions

1 /2 green pepper

1 whole roasted red pepper (jarred)

Handful black olives

1 tablespoon rosemary

Pinch ground black pepper

Pinch sea salt

INSTRUCTIONS

1. Preheat oven to 425 degrees F. Heat medium skillet to medium heat and lightly coat with coconut oil. Coat 8 or 9-inch round cake pan with coconut oil and dust with coconut flour.

2. Combine all *Crust* ingredients in small bowl. If too soft, add 1 tablespoon of coconut flour at a time. If too firm, add 1 tablespoon of water at a time. Adjust until firm dough that can hold its shape forms.

3. Form dough into ball and place in cake pan. Gently pat it into 1/4 inch thick circle, building up around edge about 1/2 - 1 inch up sides of pan. Bake crust for 5 minutes.

4. Chop sausage and rosemary. Seed and stem green pepper and peel onion. Slice onion and pepper and add to skillet with sausage. Sauté about 2 minutes.

5. Whisk eggs in medium bowl and add eggs to skillet, plus rosemary. Remove skillet from heat and scramble very lightly.

6. Reduce oven to 350 degrees F and remove pan. Carefully pour runny scrambled eggs into crust. Slice roasted red pepper and olives and sprinkle over eggs. Salt and pepper to taste.

7. Return pizza to oven and bake another 10 - 15 minutes or until eggs firm.

8. Slice and serve hot from pan. Or remove, slice and serve.

Turkey Bacon Club Salad

Prep Time: 10 minutes

Cook Time: 5 minutes

Servings: 1

INGREDIENTS

Salad:

4 slices turkey bacon

1 tablespoon coconut oil

1 heart of romaine lettuce

2 medium tomatoes, chopped

Dressing:

1 avocado

1/2 small white onion

1 small garlic clove

Juice of 1 lemon

Small bunch of parsley leaves

Pinch sea salt

Pinch ground black pepper

INSTRUCTIONS

1. Heat medium skillet to medium-high heat and add coconut oil.
2. Chop turkey bacon and add to skillet. Browned for 2 - 3 minutes on each side, until thoroughly cooked. Remove turkey bacon and preserve any leftover oil.

3. Rinse and dry heart of romaine, then chop. Dice tomato and toss with lettuce in large bowl.

4. For *Dressing*, slice avocado in half, pit, and spoon flesh into food processor or bullet blender. Add peeled onion and garlic, lemon juice and parsley. Add excess coconut oil from pan. Process until smooth. Salt and pepper to taste.

5. Use tongs to transfer lettuce and tomatoes to plate. Sprinkle on turkey bacon, and drizzle with avocado *Dressing*. Serve immediately.

Cobb Salad

Prep Time: 10 minutes

Cook Time: 10 minutes

Servings: 1

INGREDIENTS

Salad:

2 slices natural ham

2 slices nitrate-free bacon

1 heart of romaine

1/2 cup watercress

1/2 cup spinach

1 medium tomato

1/2 avocado

1 egg

Dressing:

2 tablespoons coconut oil

1 tablespoon apple cider vinegar

1 tablespoon lime juice

1 teaspoon organic mustard (or powder)

1/2 avocado

1 small clove garlic,

Small bunch cilantro

Pinch sea salt

Pinch ground black pepper

Pinch paprika

Pinch cayenne pepper

INSTRUCTIONS

1. Bring small pot to boil with salted water. Heat medium skillet over medium-high heat.

2. Gently add whole egg to boiling water for about 7 minutes, or until hard boiled.

3. While egg cooks, chop bacon and ham. Add bacon pieces to skillet. Brown bacon for about 5 minutes, until crisp and cooked on both sides. Drain bacon on paper towel. Add ham to skillet just to warm, and remove skillet from heat. Stir to warm evenly.

4. Rinse and dry heart of romaine, spinach and watercress. Chop lettuce.

5. Dice tomato. Slice in half, pit and dice flesh of half of avocado. Reserve other half.

6. Drain warm ham on paper towel. Reserve leftover bacon grease.

7. Drain hardboiled egg and cool under running water for about 30 seconds. Peel egg and chop.

8. Peel onion and garlic. Then add all *Dressing* ingredients with reserved avocado half to food processor or bullet blender. Add reserved bacon grease (optional). Process until smooth. Salt, pepper, paprika and cayenne to taste.

9. Use tongs to plate lettuce mix. Drizzle salad with avocado *Dressing*. Add chopped tomato, eggs, bacon, ham and avocado in single adjacent lines across lettuce mix. Serve immediately.

Crab Cakes

Prep Time: 5 minutes

Cook Time: 10 minutes

Servings: 2

INGREDIENTS

8 oz pre-cooked lump crabmeat

1 egg

1 lemon

1 teaspoon ground crab boil seasoning (Old Bay Seasoning™)

1 tablespoons fresh basil

1 tablespoon fresh parsley

1/4 cup almond meal

1 ripe avocado

Coconut oil (for cooking)

1. Heat large skillet over medium-high heat and coat with coconut oil.
2. Slice in half, pit and scoop flesh of half of avocado into medium mixing bowl. Preserve other half.
3. Chop basil and parsley and add to avocado. Zest lemon into bowl to taste. Cut lemon in 1/2 and squeeze about 1 tablespoon of juice into bowl, excluding seeds. Mash well.
4. Add egg to bowl blend. Add crabmeat, crab boil seasoning and almond meal. Mix gently but thoroughly.

5. Form 4 small or 2 large crabmeat patties, pressing firmly to help hold them together. They will be delicate.
6. Add crab patties to hot oiled for about 3 - 4 minutes. Carefully flip and continue cooking for another 3 - 4 minutes on each side, or until golden brown.
7. Drain crab cakes on paper towel. Slice reserved avocado. Plate crab cakes and top with sliced avocado. Drizzle with squeeze of lemon. Serve hot.

No-Oats Oatmeal

Prep Time: 5 minutes

Cook Time: 10 minutes

Servings: 2

INGREDIENTS

2 cups coconut milk

1/2 cup quick tapioca

1/4 cup chia seed

1/2 cup dried dates

1 small banana

2 tablespoons slivered almonds

2 tablespoons pumpkin seeds

2 tablespoons flaked coconut

2 tablespoons walnuts

1 tablespoon vanilla

1 teaspoon ground cinnamon

2 tablespoons raw agave nectar (optional)

Pinch sea salt

Water

INSTRUCTIONS

1. Heat medium pan over medium heat .
2. Add almonds, pumpkin seeds, coconut flakes and walnuts to hot dry pan. Dry toast about 2 minutes, stirring frequently to prevent burning.

3. Pit and chop dates. Cut banana in half and blend with coconut milk and dates in food processor or bullet blender. Reserve other half of banana.

4. Add milk mixture to hot pan. Add quick tapioca, chia seeds, vanilla and pinch of salt. Stir and thicken over heat about 5 - 8 minutes, or until tapioca is soft. Add water to loosen for runnier "oatmeal."

5. Slice reserved half of banana. Serve hot in bowl. Top with banana slices, sprinkle with cinnamon, and drizzle with agave (optional).

Acorn Squash 'N Eggs

Prep Time: 5 minutes

Cook Time: 15 minutes

Servings: 2

INGREDIENTS

1 medium acorn squash

2 eggs

1/2 small sweet onion

Ground black pepper, to taste

sea salt, to taste

1 tablespoon apple cider vinegar

Pinch of cinnamon (optional)

Coconut oil (for cooking)

INSTRUCTIONS

1. Heat large skillet over medium heat and coat generously with coconut oil. Bring medium pot to simmer with salted water, plus apple cider vinegar.

2. Peel acorn squash and onion, and grate. Drain shreddings in paper towel, pressing out moisture.

3. Combine squash, onion, black pepper and salt in small bowl. Place 4 handfuls into hot well-oiled skillet. Spread lightly to create thin, crisp patties. Brown acorn hash patties for about 5 minutes, then carefully flip. Brown another few minutes until cooked through.

4. While squash finishes, gently crack 1 egg into simmering water. Let poach for about 1 minute, then scoop out with slotted spoon and carefully drain on paper towel, careful to keep yolk intact. Repeat with second egg.

5. Plate acorn patties, 2 per person. Sprinkle with cinnamon (optional). Top with lightly poached egg. Remove from heat and serve.

Beef and Plantain Stir-Fry

Prep Time: 10 minutes

Cook Time: 15 minutes

Servings: 2

INGREDIENTS

8 oz grass-fed beef

1 sweet plantain

1 small yellow onion

1/2 red bell pepper

2 cloves garlic

1 Serrano pepper

1 teaspoon ground cumin

1 teaspoon chili powder

1 teaspoon paprika

Small bunch fresh cilantro

1/2 lime

Coconut oil (for cooking)

INSTRUCTIONS

1. Bring a medium pot to boil with lightly salted water. Leave enough room in pot for sweet plantain. Heat large skillet over high medium heat and coat with coconut oil.

2. To peel plantain, cut in half then careful make at least 4 slices through peel lengthwise. Get finger or butter knife under tough peel and pry off.

3. Cut peeled plantain cut into 1 inch pieces, then in half, forming half moons. Add to boiling water for about 5 - 8 minutes, or until tender but not mushy.

4. Stem and seed peppers. Peel onion and garlic. Dice beef into half inch cubes and add to medium bowl. Mince Serrano pepper and garlic, and add to beef. Sprinkle with cumin, chili powder and paprika. Mix with wooden spoon to avoid getting hot pepper oil on skin.

5. Slice onion and bell pepper and add to hot skillet. Sauté about 1 minute. Add seasoned beef to skillet. Sauté another 2 minutes to brown.

6. Remove plantains from boiling water and drain. Add to hot skillet and stir-fry all together for about 2 - 3 minutes, until beef is browned and cook to about medium-well and plantains are a bit caramelized.

7. Chop fresh cilantro. Remove skillet from heat and toss stir-fry with cilantro. Plate stir-fry and squeeze over lime juice. Serve hot.

Tuna Spread

Prep Time: 5 minutes

Servings: 1

INGREDIENTS

7oz (1 can) chunk light tuna

1 avocado

1/2 small red Onion

1 carrot

1 celery stalk

1/2 Lemon

1/2 cucumber

Ground black pepper, to taste

sea salt, to taste

Paprika, to taste

INSTRUCTIONS

1. Drain tuna. Cut celery stalk in half, and preserve larger end. Peel onion. Slice avocado in half, pit and scoop out flesh into small bowl. Mash well.

2. Finely dice onion, smaller half of celery stalk, and carrot. Add to bowl, with spices to taste.

3. Add tuna to bowl, plus squeeze of lemon. Mix until combined and smooth.

4. Slice reserved half of celery stalk into sticks. Slice cucumber into 1/3 inch round.

5. Serve tuna in bowl with cucumber chips and celery sticks.

Egg In A Hole

Prep Time: 5 minutes

Cook Time: 15 minutes

Servings: 2

INGREDIENTS

Pancakes:

1 3/4 cups almond meal

3/4 cup almond milk

2 eggs

1 teaspoon baking powder

1 teaspoon vanilla

Pinch sea salt

Pinch ground black pepper

Agave nectar (optional)

Coconut oil (for cooking)

Filling:

4 eggs

INSTRUCTIONS

1. Heat large skillet with lid over medium heat and lightly coat with coconut oil.
2. Whisk together 2 eggs, almond milk and vanilla in medium bowl. Whisk in almond flour, baking powder and salt until smooth.

3. Use ladle or dry measure cup to pour 1/3 of batter onto hot oiled skillet in a circle with a hole large enough for one egg. Fit up to 2 pancakes comfortably, so they do not touch as they spread.

4. Crack one egg into each space within pancake. Cover with lid and cook until sides of pancakes are firm and batter bubbles up a bit. About 3 - 4 minutes.

5. Remove lid and gently flip pancakes with spatula, careful to keep yolks intact. Cook uncovered for about 3 minutes, or until pancakes are cooked through.

6. Repeat with remaining batter. Re-oil pan if necessary. Pancakes will be slightly delicate, so flip and plate with care.

7. Sprinkle egg with salt and pepper to taste. Drizzle with agave nectar (optional). Serve warm.

Apple Nut Bake

Prep Time: 5 minutes

Cook Time: 15 minutes

Servings: 2

INGREDIENTS

Filling:

2 sweet apples

2 tart apples

2 tablespoons almond flour

2 tablespoons flax meal

1 tablespoon sweetener*

1 tablespoons ground cinnamon

1 teaspoon ground nutmeg

1 teaspoon ground ginger

1 teaspoon vanilla

Pinch sea salt

Pinch ground black pepper

Topping:

2 tablespoons coconut oil

1/2 cup almonds

1/2 cup pecans

1/2 cup walnuts

1 tablespoon ground cinnamon

1 teaspoon ground nutmeg

1 tablespoon sweetener*

Pinch sea salt

Pinch ground black pepper

INSTRUCTIONS

1. Preheat oven to 400 degrees F and lightly oil square baking pan.

2. Peel, core and dice apples. Toss apples with all *Filling* ingredients in medium bowl. Pour into baking pan.

3. Process all *Topping* ingredients in food processor or bullet blender until crumbly. Sprinkle evenly over apples.

4. Bake 15 - 20 minutes, or until apples are soft and crust is crisp. Serve hot.

*stevia, raw honey, or agave nectar

Bacon & Fruit Scramble

Prep Time: 10 minutes

Cook Time: 15 minutes

Servings: 2

INGREDIENTS

6 eggs

4 slices nitrate-free bacon

2 dried figs

1 sweet apple

1 bell pepper

1 small sweet onion

1/2 teaspoon ground black pepper

1/2 teaspoon paprika

1/2 teaspoon sea salt

1/2 teaspoon cinnamon (optional)

INSTRUCTIONS

1. Bring small pot to boil with lightly salted water. Heat medium skillet over medium-high heat.

2. Dice bacon and add to hot skillet. Brown bacon for about 3 minutes, stirring occasionally with wooden spatula.

3. Add figs to boiling water for 5 minutes.

4. Peel and core apple. Stem and seed pepper. Peel onion. Dice apple, pepper and onion and add to skillet. Sauté another 2 minutes, until veggies caramelize and bacon crisps.

5. Remove figs from boiling water and dice. Add to skillet, plus spices. Sauté another minute.

6. Crack eggs directly into skillet and scramble gently with wooden spatula.

7. Cook eggs to desired firmness and serve hot.

Salmon & Veggie Breakfast Salad

Prep Time: 10 minutes

Cook Time: 10 minutes

Servings: 1

INGREDIENTS

Salad:

1 medium salmon fillet (or 2 oz smoked salmon, do not cook)

1 carrot

1/2 cucumber

8 asparagus stalks

1 cup cabbage

1/2 lemon

Dressing:

1 avocado

2 tablespoons coconut oil

1/2 lemon

1 small clove garlic

1 tablespoon fresh parsley

1 tablespoon fresh dill

Pinch sea salt

Pinch ground black pepper

Pinch paprika

INSTRUCTIONS

1. Bring small pot to boil with salted water. Heat small skillet over medium-high heat and lightly coat with coconut oil.

2. Parboil asparagus spears in boiling water for about 2 minutes. Then drain and shock in ice bath.

3. Lay salmon fillet skin-side down in hot oiled skillet. Cook about 3 minutes on each side. Season to taste, then squeeze lemon juice over fillet.

4. Shred or grate cabbage, carrot and cucumber. Drain cucumber in paper towel. Dry asparagus in paper towel and slice into 2 inch pieces. Toss veggies together.

5. Peel garlic and add all *Dressing* ingredients with squeeze of lemon and salt, pepper and paprika to taste to food processor or bullet blender. Process until smooth.

6. Plate shredded veggies. Remove salmon fillet and flake off meat over shredded veggies. Or lay smoked salmon slices over veggies.

7. Drizzle salad with avocado *Dressing*. Squeeze a little more lemon juice over salad. Serve immediately.

Cowboy Breakfast Skillet

Prep Time: 5 minutes

Cook Time: 15 minutes

Servings: 2

INGREDIENTS

6 eggs

8 oz ground pork sausage

1 medium sweet potato

1 bell pepper

1 small red onion

Ground black pepper, to taste

Paprika, to taste

sea salt, to taste

Pinch of cinnamon (optional)

INSTRUCTIONS

1. Bring medium pot to boil with lightly salted water. Leave enough room in pot for sweet potato. Heat large skillet over medium-high heat.

2. Peel and dice sweet potato. Add to boiling water for 5 minutes.

3. Add sausage to hot skillet. Brown sausage for 5 minutes, stirring occasionally with wooden spatula.

4. While potatoes and sausage cook, seed and vein bell pepper and peel onion, then dice.

5. Beat eggs with spices in medium bowl with hand mixer or whisk.

6. Once browned, add pepper and onion to sausage. Sauté about 2 minutes, until vegetables are tender and a bit caramelized.

7. Drain sweet potatoes in colander and add to skillet. Sauté about 1 minute, until any excess liquid is evaporated. Then pour in egg mixture.

8. Scramble eggs with wooden spatula. Reduce skillet to medium heat to cook eggs evenly and avoid browning.

9. Cook and stir eggs until desired firmness. Remove from heat and serve.

Creole Frittata

Prep Time: 5 minutes

Cook Time: 15 minutes

Servings: 4

INGREDIENTS

4 Andouille sausage links

12 eggs

1 green bell pepper

1 red bell pepper

1 medium sweet onion

2 tablespoons paprika

1 teaspoon cayenne pepper

1 teaspoon onion powder

1 teaspoon garlic powder

1 teaspoon dried oregano

1 teaspoon dried thyme

1 teaspoon dried basil

1 teaspoon black pepper

1 tablespoon sea salt

Coconut oil (for cooking)

INSTRUCTIONS

1. Lightly coat large cast iron skillet with lid with coconut oil and heat over medium-high heat.

2. Cut sausage links on bias into 1/2 inch slices. Add to hot skillet.

3. While sausage browns, stem and seed peppers, and peel onion. Cut onions and peppers in half, then into 1/4 inch slices. Add to skillet and stir with wooden spatula. Sauté about 2 minutes.

4. Beat eggs with spices in large bowl with hand mixer or whisk.

5. Add eggs to browned sausage and softened veggies.

6. Reduce skillet to medium-low heat and cover with well fitting lid. Cook for about 10 minutes.

7. When eggs are firm throughout, remove from heat. Slice and serve.

Coconut and Banana Pancakes

Prep Time: 5 minutes

Cook Time: 15 minutes

Servings: 2

INGREDIENTS

Pancakes:

1 3/4 cups almond meal

1 teaspoon baking powder

2 eggs

3/4 cup coconut milk

1/4 cup flaked coconut

1/2 banana

1 teaspoon vanilla

1/4 teaspoon sea salt

Coconut oil (for cooking)

Topping:

1/2 banana

Agave nectar (optional)

INSTRUCTIONS

1. Heat a large skillet over medium-high heat and lightly coat with coconut oil.

2. Mash 1/2 banana in medium bowl with fork. Whisk in eggs, then coconut milk and vanilla.

3. Add almond flour, salt and baking powder. Whisk until smooth. Fold in coconut flakes.

4. Use ladle or dry measure cup to pour 1/4 cup of batter onto hot oiled skillet. Fit 2 or 3 pancakes comfortably, so they do not touch as they spread.

5. Cook until sides of pancakes are firm and batter bubbles up a bit. About 3 to 4 minutes.

6. Carefully flip pancakes with spatula and cook for additional minute, or until cooked through. Repeat with remaining batter. Re-oil pan if necessary. Pancakes will be slightly delicate, so flip and plate with care.

7. Slice 1/2 banana. Top with banana slices and agave nectar. Serve warm.

Pumpkin & Bacon Pancakes

Prep Time: 5 minutes

Cook Time: 15 minutes

Servings: 2

INGREDIENTS

1 3/4 cups almond flour

1 cup almond milk

1/2 cup pumpkin puree

2 eggs

1 teaspoon baking powder

2 teaspoons ground cinnamon

1 teaspoon vanilla

1/4 teaspoon sea salt

4 slices nitrate-free bacon

INSTRUCTIONS

1. Heat large skillet over high heat.
2. Chop bacon into 1/2 inch pieces. Add to hot skillet and brown. Stir occasionally with wooden spoon.
3. Whisk eggs in medium bowl. Then whisk in almond milk, pumpkin puree, vanilla and cinnamon.
4. Add almond flour, salt and baking powder. Whisk until smooth.
5. Once crisp, reduce pan to medium heat and remove bacon from pan, leaving drippings. Drain bacon bits on paper towel, then stir into pancake mixture.

6. Use ladle or dry measure cup to pour 1/4 cup of batter onto hot oiled skillet. Fit 2 or 3 pancakes comfortably, so they do not touch as they spread.

7. Cook until sides of pancakes are firm and batter bubbles up a bit. About 3 to 4 minutes.

8. Carefully flip pancakes with spatula and cook for additional minute, or until cooked through. Repeat with remaining batter. Pancakes will be slightly delicate, so flip and plate with care.

9. Serve warm. Top with topping of choice.

Tapioca Blueberry Crepes

Prep Time: 5 minutes

Cook Time: 15 minutes

Servings: 2

INGREDIENTS

Crêpes:

1 cup tapioca flour/starch

1 cup coconut milk

1 egg

Pinch sea salt

Coconut oil (for cooking)

Filling:

1 pint blueberries

2 tablespoons sweetener*

1 teaspoon vanilla

Pinch ground black pepper

Pinch sea salt

1 tablespoon water

Topping:

1/2 cup coconut crème

2 tablespoons agave nectar

1/2 teaspoon vanilla

Coconut milk (for thinning)

INSTRUCTIONS

1. Heat large non-stick pan over medium heat. Add small dollop of coconut oil and carefully spread with wadded paper towel to coat evenly . Preserve paper towel.

2. Heat medium pan over medium heat. Add all **Filling** ingredients except water. Stir occasionally with wooden spoon. Add extra tablespoon of water if blueberries do not break down enough. Remove from heat when sufficiently warmed and saucy.

3. Combine all **Crêpe** ingredients in a medium bowl. Blend thoroughly.

4. When large non-stick pan is hot, use ladle or dry measure cup to pour in 1/3 cup of crêpe batter while tilting pan in all directions to evenly spread batter.

5. Cook crêpe about 2 minutes, then carefully flip and cook another 1 - 2 minutes.

6. When both sides are lightly browned, remove crêpe to plate and oil pan with wadded paper towel. Repeat process of cooking crêpe and oiling pan with remaining batter.

7. Blend all **Topping** ingredients. Thin with small amount of coconut milk to create drizzling consistency if necessary.

8. Fill crêpes with blueberry compote down center and fold over each side. Plate fold-side down and drizzle on coconut crème **Topping**. Serve warm.

*stevia, raw honey, or agave nectar

Cashew Belgian Waffles

Prep Time: 10 minutes

Cook Time: 10 minutes

Servings: 2

INGREDIENTS

Waffles:

1 cup cashew flour (or finely ground raw cashews)

1/4 coconut flour

3 eggs, separated

1/4 cup coconut oil

4 tablespoons sweetener

1 tablespoon aluminum-free baking soda

1 teaspoon vanilla

1 pinch sea salt

1 teaspoon ground cinnamon (optional)

Topping:

1 cup fresh fruit

1/2 teaspoon vanilla

2 tablespoons water

1 tablespoon sweetener*

DIRECTIONS

1. Preheat waffle iron. Use wadded paper towel to carefully coat with coconut oil.

2. Combine flours, salt and baking soda in small bowl. In large bowl, whisk together egg yolks, oil, vanilla, plus sweetener and cinnamon (optional).

3. In separate bowl, beat egg whites to medium-stiff peaks with hand mixer. Stir flour mixture into the egg yolk mixture. Gently fold egg whites into batter.

4. Pour portion of batter onto hot waffle iron. Cook 4 - 5 minutes, until golden brown and crisp. Repeat with remain batter

5. While waffles are cooking, combine all *Topping* ingredients in small pan. Cook over stovetop until reduced and thick.

6. Top waffles with fruit compote or agave syrup (optional). Serve hot.

stevia, raw honey, or agave nectar

Apple Upside Down Cakes

Prep Time: 5 minutes

Cook Time: 15 minutes

Servings: 2

INGREDIENTS

1 3/4 cups almond meal

2 eggs

3/4 cup almond milk

2 tablespoons sweetener*

1 teaspoon baking powder

Juice of 1/2 lemon

1 teaspoon vanilla

1 teaspoon ground cinnamon

1 teaspoon ground nutmeg

1/4 teaspoon salt

1 tart apple

1/2 cup crushed pecans

INSTRUCTIONS

1. Heat large skillet over medium-high heat and lightly coat with coconut oil.
2. In medium bowl combine lemon juice, vanilla, cinnamon and nutmeg.
3. Peel and core apple, then slice in half length-wise. Lay halves down on flat side and slice thinly from top of apple to bottom.

Carefully toss apple slices in lemon juice and spices. Try not to break any.

4. Arrange apple slices into a circle by overlapping at the bottom and fanning out. Try to make at least 4 circles.

5. Add eggs and almond milk into leftover lemon juice and spices and whisk until combined. Add almond flour, salt and baking powder. Whisk until smooth.

6. Use oiled spatula to lift apples, keeping their arrangement, and place into hot pan. Get at least two apple arrangements into pan together. Sprinkle chopped pecans into pan around apple circles.

7. Use ladle or dry measure cup to pour 1/3 cup of batter over and around apple arrangements in skillet. Do not let pancakes touch as they spread.

8. Cook until sides of pancakes are firm and batter bubbles up a bit. About 3 - 4 minutes.

9. Flip pancakes with spatula, careful not to disturb apples. Cook for additional minute, or until cooked through. Repeat with remaining batter. Re-oil pan if necessary.

10. Pancakes will be slightly delicate, so flip and plate with care.

11. Sprinkle with cinnamon. Serve warm.

*stevia, raw honey, or agave nectar

Lunch Recipes

Chicken Fries with Garlic Aioli
Chicken Noodle Soup
Simple Gazpacho + Tortilla Chips
Sweet Potato Fries + Ketchup
Oyster Po' Boy
Sausage And Peppers Sub
Tuna Sandwich
Crispy Fish Sandwich with Quick Slaw
Kelp Noodle Stir-Fry
Shrimp Taco
Spicy Mango Fried Rice
Quick Chili
Seared Tuna Salad
Chimichangas
Soft Burger Buns
Long Rolls
Sandwich Bread
Soft Baked Pita
Grain-Free Tortillas
BBQ Pork Sandwich
California Turkey Burger
BLT
Chicken Souvlaki + Tzatziki

Gyro + Avocado Tzatziki
Meatball Sub
Cheese Steak Sandwich
Veggie Burger
Crisp Spinach Salad
Egg Salad Sandwich
Kelp Noodle Salad

Chicken Fries with Garlic Aioli

Prep Time: 10 minutes

Cook Time: 15 minutes

Servings: 2

INGREDIENTS

8 oz boneless, skinless chicken breast

1 egg

1/2 cup almond meal

1 teaspoon flax meal (or ground chia seed)

1 teaspoon ground black pepper

1/2 teaspoon paprika

1/2 teaspoon onion powder

1/2 teaspoon garlic powder

1/2 teaspoon chili powder

1/2 teaspoon sea salt

Garlic Aioli

1/2 - 3/4 cup coconut oil

1 egg yolk

2 garlic cloves

1/2 small lemon

1/4 teaspoon ground white pepper (or black pepper)

1/4 teaspoon sea salt

3 tablespoons flavorful oil (black truffle, walnut, almond, sesame, etc.)

(optional)

INSTRUCTIONS

1. Heat large pan over medium-high heat and coat with coconut oil.

2. For *Garlic Aioli*, peel garlic and add to food processor or blender with egg yolk, juice of 1/2 lemon, salt and pepper. Process until smooth, scraping down sides of vessel.

3. While processor or blender is running, very slowly drizzle in enough coconut oil to create thick mayo-like mixture. Drizzle in flavorful oil as well will processor runs (optional). If mixture is runny, drizzle in more coconut oil while processor runs until thickened. Pour into serving dish and refrigerate.

4. Slice chicken into half width-wise, creating twice the fillets. Try to slice at thickest portion to keep all fillets equal thickness.

5. Slice chicken fillets into long, 1/2 inch wide strips. Place strips between two paper towels and press to absorb excess moisture.

6. In a shallow dish, blend almond meal, flax or chia meal, spices and salt.

7. Beat egg in small mixing bowl. Toss chicken strips in beaten egg to lightly coat, then dredge in seasoned almond meal.

8. Carefully place coated chicken strips into hot oil and fry about 2 - 3 minutes, until golden brown and cooked through. Turn with tongs half way through cooking.

9. Drain cooked chicken on paper towel, then transfer to serving dish.

10. Serve hot with *Garlic Aioli*.

Chicken Noodle Soup

Prep Time: 10 minutes

Cook Time: 20 minutes

Servings: 2

INGREDIENTS

Noodles

1/2 cup almond flour

1/2 cup arrowroot powder

1/2 cup tapioca flour

1 egg

2 egg yolks

1 tablespoon coconut oil

1/2 teaspoon sea salt

Soup

8 oz skin-on chicken

1 1/2 cup chicken broth or stock

1/2 cup water

2 carrots

1 celery stalk

2 teaspoons dried thyme (4 teaspoons fresh thyme)

1/2 teaspoon black pepper

Pinch sea salt

INSTRUCTIONS

1. Heat medium pot over medium-high heat. Place chicken skin-side down in hot pot. Sear and render out fat for about 5 minutes.
2. Dice carrots and celery. Add to chicken with salt and pepper.
3. Turn chicken and brown on flesh side about 5 minutes. Stir veggies as well.
4. Add thyme, chicken stock and water, and increase heat to high. Bring soup to simmer. Adjust heat as necessary and keep at simmer or soft boil.
5. For *Noodles*, sift almond flour, tapioca flour, 1/3 cup arrow powder and salt into medium mixing bowl. Make well in the center of flour mixture and add egg and yolks. Whisk eggs into flour in circular motion with a fork until dough pulls together.
6. Dust cutting board with half of remaining arrowroot powder. Turn dough out onto cutting board and knead for 5 minutes, until smooth.
7. Add 1 tablespoon coconut oil if dough is too dry. Add 1 tablespoon almond flour at a time if dough is too moist or sticky.
8. Dust cutting board with remaining arrowroot powder. Roll dough into rectangular shape with a rolling pin to about 1/8 inch thickness. Cut pasta sheet into long strips with pizza cutter or sharp knife. Or run past through pasta machine several times until desired thickness is reached. Then use cutting attachment to cut pasta into preferred style.
9. Separate noodles a bit and place gently in simmering soup for about 3 minutes.
10. Transfer to serving dish and serve immediately.

Simple Gazpacho + Tortilla Chips

Prep Time: 20 minutes

Cook Time: 10 minutes

Servings: 4

INGREDIENTS

Grain-Free Tortillas

Gazpacho

2 (11.5 oz) cans organic tomato juice (or 3 cups juiced tomatoes)

4 plum tomatoes

2 red bell peppers

1 red onion

1 cucumber

3 garlic cloves

1/4 cup apple cider vinegar

1/4 cup coconut oil (or 2 tablespoons coconut oil and 2 tablespoons flavorful oil [walnut, almond, sesame, etc.])

1 teaspoon cracked black pepper (or ground black pepper)

1/2 tablespoon sea salt

INSTRUCTIONS

1. Seed cucumber and tomatoes. Seed, stem and vein bell peppers. Peel onion and garlic. Dice veggies, mince garlic, and add to medium serving bowl.

2. Add tomato juice, vinegar, oil, salt and pepper, and mix well. Place in refrigerator.

3. Heat medium pan over medium-high heat and coat with coconut oil.

4. For *Tortilla Chips*, prepare *Grain-Free Tortillas*.

5. Add more coconut oil to hot pan and allow to heat up. Cut tortillas into wedges with pizza cutter or sharp knife.

6. Add tortilla wedges back to hot pan in single layer and cook about 30 seconds on each side, until golden and crisp. Drain on paper towel. Repeat with remaining tortilla wedges.

7. Transfer warm *Tortilla Chips* to serving dish. Serve immediately with chilled *Gazpacho*.

Sweet Potato Fries + Ketchup

Prep Time: 5 minutes

Cook Time: 35 minutes

Servings: 2

INGREDIENTS

Sweet Potato Fries

1 large sweet potato

2 tablespoons coconut oil

1/2 teaspoon ground black pepper

1/2 teaspoon ground paprika

1/2 teaspoon sea salt

1/4 teaspoon cayenne pepper (optional)

Ketchup

4 oz (1/2 can) organic tomato sauce

6 oz (1 can) organic tomato paste

1 tablespoon apple cider vinegar

1/2 teaspoon garlic powder

1/2 teaspoon onion powder

1/2 teaspoon ground black pepper

INSTRUCTIONS

1. Preheat oven to 450 degrees F. Line sheet pan with parchment or coat lightly with coconut oil.
2. Peel sweet potato if preferred, but do not rinse. Slice sweet potato into 1/4 inch strips and add to medium mixing bowl with coconut

oil, black pepper, paprika and cayenne (optional). Toss potatoes until well coated.

3. Spread fries in well-spaced, single layer on sheet pan. Sprinkle salt over potatoes.

4. Place sheet pan in oven and bake for 10 minutes.

5. Carefully remove sheet pan and turn fries over with tongs or spatula. Place sheet pan bake into oven. Bake for another 10 minutes, or until golden and crispy.

6. While *Sweet Potato Fries* bake, add tomato sauce, tomato paste, vinegar, garlic powder, onion powder and black pepper to small pot.

7. Heat pot over medium heat and reduced for about 5 minutes, stirring occasionally.

8. Once reduced, remove pot from heat. Transfer ketchup to serving dish and refrigerate about 20 minutes.

9. Remove sheet pan from oven and serve *Sweet Potato Fries* hot with *Ketchup*.

Oyster Po' Boy

Prep Time: 15 minutes

Cook Time: 20 minutes

Servings: 2

INGREDIENTS

Long Rolls

12 oysters

1/2 cup coconut flour

1 egg

1 avocado

1 tablespoon lemon juice

1 sprig fresh dill

1 rib lettuce

1 small tomato

8 - 12 dill pickle chips

1/2 teaspoon black pepper

1/2 teaspoon salt

Coconut oil (for cooking)

INSTRUCTIONS

1. Preheat oven to 350 degrees F. Line sheet pan with parchment paper, or lightly coat with coconut oil. Or lightly coat 6 mini loaf pans with coconut oil.
2. Prepare *Long Rolls* and place in oven.
3. Heat small pan over medium heat. Coat with coconut oil.

4. Add coconut flour to small bowl. Beat egg with salt and pepper in separate mixing bowl. Dip each oyster in beaten egg, then dredge in coconut flour.

5. Place each oyster in hot oiled pan and cook until crispy and lightly browned, about 2 minutes on each side.

6. Remove oysters from pan and drain on paper towels.

7. Finely mince dill. Slice and pit avocado. Scoop flesh into small bowl and mix with lemon juice and dill until smooth. Shred lettuce and slice tomatoes.

8. Remove *Long Rolls* from oven and let cool about 2 minutes.

9. Slice rolls along side and spread with avocado mixture. Place shredded lettuce on bottom of bun, then add 6 fried oysters. Top with tomato slices and pickles.

10. Serve immediately.

Sausage And Peppers Sub

Prep Time: 20 minutes

Cook Time: 20 minutes

Servings: 4

INSTRUCTIONS

Long Rolls

4 Italian sausage links (pork, chicken, etc.)

1 yellow onion

1 green bell pepper

DIRECTIONS

1. Preheat oven to 350 degrees F. Line sheet pan with parchment paper, or lightly coat with coconut oil. Or lightly coat 6 mini loaf pans with coconut oil.
2. Prepare *Long Rolls* and place in oven.
3. Heat medium skillet over medium heat.
4. Add sausage to hot skillet and sear about 8 minutes.
5. Peel onion, and stem and seed bell pepper. Slice onion and pepper and add to skillet. Stir and sauté veggies.
6. Cooked sausage and veggies about 8 minutes, until sausage is cooked through and veggies are tender and caramelized.
7. Remove *Long Rolls* from oven and let cool about 2 minutes.
8. Slice rolls along side or split through top. Place cooked sausage on roll and top with peppers and onions.
9. Serve hot.

Tuna Sandwich

Prep Time: 10 minutes

Cook Time: 15 minutes

Servings: 1

INSTRUCTIONS

Sandwich Bread

7 oz (1 can) chunk light tuna

1/2 avocado

1/2 small red onion

1 small carrot

1 small celery stalk

1/2 small cucumber

1/2 lemon

1/2 teaspoon paprika

1/4 teaspoon cracked black pepper (or ground black pepper)

1/4 teaspoon sea salt

DIRECTIONS

1. Preheat oven to 350 degrees F. Lightly coat 6 mini round cake pans or medium loaf pan with coconut oil. Bring medium pot of lightly salted water to a boil.
2. Prepare *Sandwich Bread* and place in oven.
3. While bread bakes, drain tuna and add to small mixing bowl. Cut celery stalk and carrot in half length-wise. Peel onion and cucumber. Finely dice celery, carrot and onion. Add to bowl.

4. Slice avocado in half and scoop flesh of non-pit half into bowl. Preserve pitted half in airtight container with pit intact for freshness.

5. Add salt, pepper paprika and squeeze of 1/2 lemon into bowl. Mash together with fork until combined and smooth. Slice cucumber into 1/4 inch rounds.

6. Refrigerate tuna mixture if preferred.

7. Remove *Sandwich Bread* from oven and let cool about 5 minutes.

8. Slice bread and fill with tuna mixture. Top with cucumber slices.

9. Serve immediately.

Crispy Fish Sandwich with Quick Slaw

Prep Time: 20 minutes

Cook Time: 20 minutes

Servings: 1

INSTRUCTIONS

Soft Burger Bun

Crispy Fish

6 oz fillet white fish (cod, tilapia, catfish, etc.)

1/4 cup almond meal

1 egg

1/2 teaspoon ground black pepper

1/2 teaspoon sea salt

Quick Slaw

1/4 head cabbage (1 cup shredded)

1 small carrot

zest of 1/2 lemon

Juice of 1/2 lemon

2 tablespoons coconut oil

1 - 2 tablespoons apple cider vinegar

1 tablespoon sweetener* (optional)

1/4 teaspoon ground white pepper (or black pepper)

1 teaspoon sea salt

DIRECTIONS

1. Preheat oven to 350 degrees F. Line sheet pan with parchment paper, or lightly coat with coconut oil. Or lightly coat 6 mini round cake pans with coconut oil.

2. Prepare *Soft Burger Buns* and place in oven.

3. While bread bakes, heat small skillet over medium heat and coat with coconut oil.

4. For *Quick Slaw*, remove any tough outer leaves and core from cabbage. Shred cabbage and carrot. Add to medium mixing bowl with vinegar, coconut oil, sweetener, salt and pepper. Zest *then* juice lemon, and add. Toss to combine and place in refrigerator.

5. For *Crispy Fish*, beat egg with half of salt and pepper in small mixing bowl. Mix almond flour with remaining salt and pepper in small dish.

6. Coat fish fillet in egg then dredge in almond flour. Place fillet in hot oiled pan and cook about 3 minutes on each side, until crispy and golden but still juicy.

7. Remove fish from pan and drain on paper towels.

8. Remove *Soft Burger Bun* from oven and let cool about 5 minutes.

9. Slice bun in half and add *Crispy Fish*. Top with *Quick Slaw* and serve immediately.

*stevia, raw honey or agave nectar

Kelp Noodle Stir-Fry

Prep Time: 10 minutes

Cook Time: 10 minutes

Servings: 2

INSTRUCTIONS

1 (12 oz) package kelp noodles

8 oz grass-fed beef

1/2 sweet onion

1 red bell pepper

1 hot chili pepper

2 cloves garlic

1 inch piece fresh ginger

1/2 teaspoon paprika

1/2 teaspoon ground black pepper

1/4 teaspoon sea salt

Small bunch fresh cilantro

1 lime

Coconut oil (for cooking)

DIRECTIONS

1. Heat large skillet or medium cast-iron wok over high heat. Drain and rinse kelp noodles. Add to medium bowl and soak for 5 minutes in water and juice of 1/2 lime.

2. Stem and seed peppers. Peel onion, garlic and ginger. Dice beef into strips and add to medium mixing bowl. Mince chili pepper,

garlic and ginger. Add to beef with salt, pepper, paprika and 1 teaspoon coconut oil. Mix with wooden spoon to evenly coat beef.

3. Slice onion and bell pepper and add to hot skillet. Sauté about 2 minutes. Add seasoned beef to skillet and sauté another 2 minutes to brown.

4. Drain kelp noodles and add to skillet. Stir until beef is browned and cooked to about medium-well, kelp noodles are heated through, and veggies caramelize.

5. Remove skillet from heat and plate stir-fry. Chop fresh cilantro.

6. Top stir-fry with cilantro and squeeze of 1/2 lime.

7. Serve hot.

Shrimp Taco

Prep Time: 15 minutes

Cook Time: 20 minutes

Servings: 4

INGREDIENTS

Grain-Free Tortillas

Filling

12 oz medium shrimp

1/2 small red onion

1 fresh jalapeño or (2 oz pickled jalapeño)

1 garlic clove

1/2 inch piece ginger root

1/4 head cabbage (1 cup shredded)

Large bunch cilantro

1 avocado

1 tomato

2 limes

Coconut oil (for cooking)

INSTRUCTIONS

1. Heat large pan over medium-high heat and lightly coat with coconut oil.
2. Prepare *Grain-Free Tortillas*, with 4 smaller portions.
3. Keep tortillas warm and moist in oven set to WARM under damp paper towel.

4. Use clean paper towel to carefully wipe out pan. Add 1 tablespoon coconut oil to pan.

5. Peel and devein shrimp, and remove tail. Peel and mince garlic and ginger. Peel and thinly slice onion. Slice fresh jalapeños.

6. Add shrimp to pan with garlic, ginger, onion and jalapeños. Sauté about 2 minutes, then squeeze juice of 1 lime and sprinkle pinch of salt and pepper over shrimp.

7. Sauté shrimp until just cooked, about 5 minutes. Remove from heat.

8. Grate radish, shred cabbage, dice tomato. Slice avocado in half, remove pit, and slice flesh in peel. Chop cilantro.

9. Remove tortillas from oven and layer with sautéed shrimp and onions. Top with shredded cabbage, radish, tomato and avocado slices. Finish with large pinch of cilantro and squeeze of lime.

10. Fold tortillas and serve warm.

Spicy Mango Fried Rice

Prep Time: 10 minutes

Cook Time: 15 minutes

Servings: 4

INGREDIENTS

1 head cauliflower

8 oz boneless, skinless chicken

1 mango

1 hot chili pepper

2 scallions

2 garlic cloves

3 tablespoons pure fish sauce (or coconut aminos)

3 teaspoons sesame oil (or walnut or almond oil)

1/2 teaspoon red pepper flake

1/2 lime

Coconut oil (for cooking)

INSTRUCTIONS

1. Heat large skillet or medium cast-iron wok over high heat. Lightly coat with coconut oil.

2. Cut cauliflower into florets and add to food processor with shredding attachment to rice. Or finely mince cauliflower.

3. Peel garlic and ginger and mince. Mince chili pepper. Thinly slice scallions. Carefully peel and dice mango. Dice chicken.

4. Add diced chicken, garlic, ginger, chili pepper and red pepper flake to hot skillet or wok. Sauté until chicken is golden brown and just cooked, about 3 minutes. Remove chicken and set aside.
5. Add cauliflower to hot pan or wok. Sauté about 5 minutes, until cauliflower is golden and a bit softened.
6. Add mango and scallions and cook another 2 - 5minutes, until cauliflower is cooked through.
7. Add chicken to cauliflower and stir.
8. Remove from heat and serve hot with a squeeze of lime.

Quick Chili

Prep Time: 5 minutes

Cook Time: 20 minutes

Servings: 4

INGREDIENTS

1 lb lean grass-fed ground beef (or elk, bison, turkey or chicken)

15 oz (1 can) organic tomato sauce

6 oz (1 can) organic tomato paste

1 small onion

1 bell pepper

2 cloves garlic

2 tablespoons chili powder

1 tablespoon ground cumin

1 tablespoon smoked paprika (or paprika)

1 teaspoon Mexican oregano (or dried oregano)

1 teaspoon ground black pepper

1 teaspoon sea salt

1/2 teaspoon cayenne pepper

1 tablespoon coconut oil

sea salt, to taste

INSTRUCTIONS

1. Heat medium pot over medium-high heat. Add 1 tablespoon coconut oil.

2. Peel onion and garlic. Stem and seed bell pepper. Chop and add to food processor or bullet blender. Pulse until finely minced.

3. Add to skillet and sauté for about 1 minute. Add ground beef and spices. Brown beef for about 5 minutes. Stir with whisk to break up meat well, or wooden spoon to keep beef chunkier.

4. Add whole cans of tomato sauce and paste. Stir to combine.

5. Bring to a simmer, then reduce heat to medium and cover loosely with lid to prevent splatter. Simmer about 10 minutes. Stir occasionally.

6. Use large serving spoon or ladle to serve hot.

Seared Tuna Salad

Prep Time: 10 minutes

Cook Time: 10 minutes

Servings: 1

INGREDIENTS

1 cup spinach

1 cup arugula

1 avocado

Seared Tuna

6 oz sushi-grade tuna steak

1 tablespoon sesame oil (or coconut oil)

Juice of 1/2 lemon

1 glove garlic

1/2 inch piece fresh ginger

1 teaspoon sesame seeds

Ginger Glaze

1/2 cup pure fish sauce (or coconut aminos)

1/4 cup apple cider vinegar

Juice of 1 1/2 lemons

2 tablespoons sweetener*

1 inch piece fresh ginger

1 green onion

INSTRUCTIONS

1. For *Ginger Glaze*, peel and grate fresh ginger and slice scallion. Add to small pot with fish sauce, vinegar, sweetener and lemon juice. Heat over medium heat and bring to a simmer. Simmer 5 - 7 minutes, until slightly reduced and thickened. Stir occasionally. Once reduced, transfer to serving dish and refrigerate.

2. For *Seared Tuna*, peel and grate or mince ginger and garlic. Add to small dish with lemon juice and sesame oil and mix to combine. Roll tuna steak in marinade to coat and let sit in dish for 10 minutes in refrigerator.

3. Slice avocado in half and pit. Slice flesh in peel. Place halves together to keep avocado from browning while continuing.

4. Heat small skillet over medium-high heat. Add 1 tablespoon coconut oil.

5. Place marinated tuna in hot oiled pan and sear on each side about 1 minute, until outer flesh is just crisped but inside *is not* cooked through. About 5 minutes.

6. Remove tuna and sprinkle with sesame seeds. Cut tuna into slices.

7. Plate spinach and arugula. Fan out avocado slices over salad.

8. Top salad with *Seared Tuna*. Drizzle on chilled *Ginger Glaze* and serve immediately.

*stevia, raw honey or agave nectar

Chimichangas

Prep Time: 20 minutes*

Cook Time: 30 minutes

Servings: 2

INGREDIENTS

Grain-Free Tortillas

Almond Cheese

1 cup skinless almonds*

1/4 cup water

2 tablespoons coconut oil

1 tablespoon lemon juice

1 tablespoon apple cider vinegar

1 garlic clove

1/2 teaspoon sea salt

1/4 teaspoon ground white pepper (or black pepper)

Filling

12 oz boneless, skinless chicken

1/2 teaspoon paprika

1/2 teaspoon ground cumin

Sauce

8 oz (1 can) organic tomato sauce

1 (canned or jarred) green chili

1/2 small white onion

5 pickled jalapeño slices

1 teaspoon ground cumin

1 teaspoon chili powder

1 teaspoon smoked paprika (or paprika)

1/2 teaspoon ground black pepper

1/2 teaspoon sea salt

Topping

Small bunch cilantro

2 ribs lettuce

1 plum tomato

1 lime

INSTRUCTIONS

1. *For *Almond Cheese,* soak almonds in enough water to cover well overnight. Drain and rinse.

2. Add all *Almond Cheese* ingredients to food processor or bullet blender and process until smooth. Add a few extra tablespoons of water if necessary to achieve thick but smooth consistency. Set aside.

3. Preheat oven to 450 degrees F. Heat medium pan over medium-high heat and coat with coconut oil.

4. Prepare *Grain-Free Tortillas.*

5. Spread 1/2 of *Almond Cheese* on tortillas and place sautéed chicken down center of each tortilla. Fold roll each tortilla into a burrito-like shape, tucking folds under.

6. Brush baking dish with coconut oil and place chimichangas in baking dish seam-side down. Place in oven and bake about 8 - 10 minutes, until golden and slightly crisp.

7. Add *Sauce* ingredients to food processor or bullet blender and process until smooth.

8. Add to small pot and heat over medium-high heat. Stir and simmer about 10 minutes until reduced and thickened. Once reduced, remove from heat.

9. Chop cilantro, shred lettuce, dice tomato and cut lime into wedges while everything cooks.

10. Remove chimichangas from oven and place on serving dish. Spread remaining *Almond Cheese* over tortillas and drizzle on *Sauce*. Top with cilantro, lettuce and tomato.

11. Squeeze on lime and serve hot with lime wedges.

Soft Burger Buns

Prep Time: 5 minutes

Cook Time: 15 minutes

Servings: 6

INGREDIENTS

1/4 cup almond flour

1/4 cup coconut flour

4 eggs

2 tablespoons coconut oil

2 tablespoons unsweetened applesauce

1 teaspoon flax meal (or ground chia seed)

1 teaspoon baking powder

1/2 teaspoon sea salt

INSTRUCTIONS

1. Preheat oven to 350 degrees F. Line sheet pan with parchment paper, or lightly coat with coconut oil. Or lightly coat 6 mini round cake pans with coconut oil.
2. Beat eggs, coconut oil and applesauce in medium mixing bowl with hand mixer or whisk.
3. In large mixing bowl, sift together coconut flour, almond flour, flax or chia meal, baking powder and salt. Pour egg mixture into flour mixture and mix until combined.
4. Scoop thick batter onto prepared sheet pan in six 4 inch rounds. Or pour into six prepared mini cake pans for uniformity. Smooth batter with knife or spatula.

5. Place in oven and bake for 12 - 15 minutes, or until tops are firm to the touch and golden.
6. Remove from oven and let cool at least 5 minutes.
7. Slice in half and serve with your favorite patty or filling.

Long Rolls

Prep Time: 5 minutes

Cook Time: 15 minutes

Servings: 6

INGREDIENTS

1/4 cup almond flour

1/4 cup coconut flour

1/4 cup full-fat coconut milk

3 eggs

2 tablespoons unsweetened applesauce

2 tablespoons tapioca flour (or arrowroot powder)

1 teaspoon baking powder

1/2 teaspoon sea salt

INSTRUCTIONS

1. Preheat oven to 350 degrees F. Line sheet pan with parchment paper, or lightly coat with coconut oil. Or lightly coat 6 mini loaf pans with coconut oil.

2. Beat eggs, coconut milk and applesauce in medium mixing bowl with hand mixer or whisk.

3. In large mixing bowl, sift together coconut flour, almond flour, tapioca or arrowroot, baking powder and salt. Pour egg mixture into flour mixture and mix until combined.

4. Scoop thick batter onto prepared sheet pan in six long forms. Or pour into six prepared mini loaf pans for uniformity. Smooth batter with knife or spatula.

5. Place in oven and bake for 12 - 15 minutes, or until golden and tops are firm to the touch.

6. Remove from oven and let cool at least 5 minutes.

7. Slice in half or split through top, and serve with your favorite link or filling.

Sandwich Bread

Prep Time: 5 minutes

Cook Time: 15 minutes

Servings: 6

INGREDIENTS

2 cups almond flour

4 eggs

1/2 cup coconut cream (or melted cacao butter)

1/2 cup arrowroot powder (or tapioca flour)

1/3 cup ground chia seed (or flax meal)

1/4 cup coconut oil

2 tablespoons unsweetened applesauce

1 teaspoon apple cider vinegar

1 teaspoon baking soda

1/2 teaspoon sea salt

INSTRUCTIONS

1. Preheat oven to 350 degrees F. Lightly coat 6 mini round cake pans with coconut oil.

2. Beat eggs, coconut oil, coconut cream, applesauce and vinegar in medium mixing bowl with hand mixer or whisk.

3. In large mixing bowl, sift together almond flour, arrowroot, chia meal, baking soda and salt. Pour egg mixture into flour mixture and mix until well combined.

4. Pour batter into prepared mini cake pans and bake for about 15 minutes, or until golden brown and toothpick inserted comes out clean.
5. Remove from oven and let cool at least 5 minutes.
6. Slice in half and serve with your favorite deli meats or sandwich salads.

NOTE: Lightly oil medium loaf pan and bake for about 25 minutes for **Sandwich Bread** loaf.

Soft Baked Pita

Prep Time: 5 minutes

Cook Time: 20 minutes

Servings: 1

INGREDIENTS

1 cup tapioca flour

1 tablespoon ground chia seed (or flax meal)

2 eggs

2 tablespoons coconut oil

1/4 cup water

1/2 teaspoon baking soda

1/4 teaspoon sea salt

INSTRUCTIONS

1. Preheat oven to 350 degrees F. Cover sheet pan with parchment paper or baking mat. Heat small pot over low heat.

2. Mix 1/3 cup tapioca flour with chia meal, water and 1 tablespoon coconut oil in pot. Stir until mixture comes together. Remove from heat and cool in freezer.

3. In medium bowl, blend remaining tapioca flour, baking soda and salt. Then beat in eggs and remaining oil with hand mixer or whisk until combined.

4. Add cooled chia mixture to egg mixture and mix to combine with wooden spoon or spatula. Remove mixture and knead to form soft dough.

5. Form large round disk and flatten on lined baking sheet with hands or rolling pin.

6. Place in oven and bake for about 10 minutes. Carefully turn over with spatula and bake another 10 minutes, or until firm.

7. Remove from oven and let cool about 5 minutes.

8. Fill with grilled meats and veggies and serve warm.

Grain-Free Tortillas

Prep Time: 5 minutes

Cook Time: 10 minutes

Servings: 2

INGREDIENTS

2 tablespoons almond flour

2 tablespoons coconut flour

1/2 tablespoon flax meal (or ground chia seed)

2 eggs

1/4 cup water (plus extra)

2 tablespoons coconut oil

1/4 teaspoon baking powder

Coconut oil (for cooking)

INSTRUCTIONS

1. Heat medium frying pan over medium-high heat and coat with coconut oil.

2. Whisk together eggs, coconut oil and 1/4 cup water in medium bowl.

3. In separate mixing bowl, blend coconut flour, almond flour, flax or chia seed, and baking powder.

4. Slowly whisk as you pour flourmixture into wet ingredients. If batter appears too thick to spread fairly thin in pan, add up to 4 tablespoon water 1 tablespoon at a time.

5. Use ladle or dry measure cup to pour 1/2 of batter into hot oiled pan. Tilt pan in circular motion as you pour so batter spreads thinly.

6. Cook batter for about 2 minutes or until slightly golden and firm. Flip tortilla with tongs or spatula and cook another 2 minutes. Remove and place on paper towel or parchment.

7. Cook remaining batter for 2 minutes on each side. Re-oil pan as necessary.

8. Fill warm tortillas with meat or veggies of choice and serve warm.

BBQ Pork Sandwich

Prep Time: 5 minutes

Cook Time: 15 minutes

Servings: 4

INGREDIENTS

Sandwich Bread

BBQ Pork

16 oz (1 lb) boneless pork (slow roasted or fresh)

8 oz (1 can) organic tomato sauce

1/2 small sweet onion

1 garlic clove

2 tablespoons sweetener*

1 tablespoon coconut oil

1 tablespoon apple cider vinegar

2 tablespoons paprika

1/2 teaspoon ground black pepper

1 teaspoon sea salt

INSTRUCTIONS

1. Preheat oven to 350 degrees F. Lightly coat 6 mini round cake pans with coconut oil. Heat medium skillet over medium-high heat and add 1 tablespoon coconut oil.
2. Prepare *Sandwich Bread* and place in oven.

3. While bread bakes, thinly slice and shred fresh pork, and add to hot oiled skillet. Or shred roasted pork with hands or fork and set aside.

4. Peel garlic and onion. Add to food processor or bullet blender with tomato sauce, sweetener, vinegar , salt and spice. Process until smooth.

5. Sauté fresh pork about 5 - 7 minutes, until browned, then add tomato mixture to pan. Or add tomato mixture to pan and reduce about 5 minutes, then add roasted pork.

6. Stir and simmer another 5 minutes, until sauce is reduce and fresh pork is cooked through, or roasted pork is heated through.

7. Remove *Sandwich Bread* from oven and let cool about 5 minutes. Slice and fill with *BBQ Pork*.

8. Serve warm.

raw honey or agave nectar

California Turkey Burger

Prep Time: 5 minutes

Cook Time: 15 minutes

Servings: 4

INGREDIENTS

Soft Burger Bun

16 - 20 oz ground turkey

4 - 6 slices nitrate free bacon

1 avocado

1 heirloom tomato

2 ribs romaine lettuce (or preferred lettuce)

1/2 cup alfalfa sprouts

sea salt, to taste

Ground black pepper, to taste

INSTRUCTIONS

1. Preheat oven to 350 degrees F. Line sheet pan with parchment paper, or lightly coat with coconut oil. Or lightly coat 6 mini round cake pans with coconut oil. Heat medium skillet over medium-high heat.
2. Prepare *Soft Burger Buns* and place in oven.
3. While bread bakes, cut bacon strips in half and place in hot pan. Cook about 5 minutes, until browned and crisp on both sides. Set bacon aside.

4. Form ground turkey into 4 patties and place in hot pan. Reduce heat to medium. Sprinkle with salt and pepper and sear 4 -5 minutes on each side.

5. Cut lettuce ribs in half. Cut tomato into 4 thick slices. Slice avocado in half, pit and slice flesh in peel.

6. Remove *Soft Burger Bun* from oven and let cool about 5 minutes.

7. Slice bun in half and place lettuce on bottom bun, followed by tomato slice. Add burger patty, then 2 - 3 bacon strip halves, and a pinch of alfalfa sprouts. Top with a few slices of avocado and top bun.

8. Serve immediately.

BLT

Prep Time: 10 minutes*

Cook Time: 20 minutes

Servings: 2

INGREDIENTS

Sandwich Bread

8 slices nitrate-free bacon

1 large tomato

2 ribs romaine lettuce

1/2 cup arugula leaves

1/2 cup baby spinach

Honey Mustard

2 oz organic mustard

2 tablespoons sweetener*

INSTRUCTIONS

1. Preheat oven to 350 degrees F. Lightly coat 6 mini round cake pans with coconut oil. Or lightly coat loaf pan with coconut oil. Heat medium skillet over medium-high heat.
2. Prepare *Sandwich Bread* and place in oven.
3. While bread bakes, cut bacon strips in half and place in hot pan. Cook about 5 minutes, until browned and crisp on both sides. Remove skillet from heat and set bacon aside.

4. Shred romaine lettuce and toss with spinach and arugula. Thinly slice tomato. Mix mustard and sweetener in small mixing bowl.

5. Remove *Sandwich Bread* from oven and let cool about 5 minutes. Slice and spread with *Honey Mustard*.

6. Layer bottom bread slice with half lettuce mix, tomato slices and crisp bacon. Top sandwich with top bread slice and cut in half on the diagonal. Repeat with second sandwich.

7. Serve immediately.

*raw honey or agave nectar

Chicken Souvlaki + Tzatziki

Prep Time: 10 minutes

Cook Time: 20 minutes

Servings: 1

INGREDIENTS

Soft Baked Pita

6 oz boneless skinless chicken

2 tablespoons fresh lemon juice

1/2 teaspoon dried oregano

2 garlic cloves

1/2 teaspoon sea salt

2 teaspoons coconut oil

1 rib romaine lettuce

1/2 tomato

1/2 small white onion

Tzatziki

1/2 small cucumber

1/4 cup coconut cream (or kefir)

1 teaspoon lemon juice

1/2 teaspoon apple cider vinegar (optional, if using coconut cream)

1 garlic clove

1/4 teaspoon salt

INSTRUCTIONS

10. Preheat oven to 350 degrees F. Cover sheet pan with parchment paper or baking mat. Heat small pot over low heat.

11. Prepare *Soft Baked Pita* and place in oven.

12. While pita bakes, peel and mince garlic. Pierce chicken multiple times with fork. Then cut chicken into one inch cubes.

13. Add chicken to small mixing bowl with lemon juice, oregano, garlic, salt and 1 teaspoon coconut oil. Let chicken marinate in refrigerator for 10 minutes.

14. For *Tzatziki*, peel, seed and shred or grate cucumber. Peel and mince garlic. Add to small mixing bowl with lemon juice, coconut cream, salt and vinegar (optional). Mix well, then place in refrigerator to chill.

15. Heat small skillet or griddle over medium-high heat and add 1 teaspoon coconut oil.

16. Drain marinated chicken and add to hot oiled skillet or griddle. Grill chicken for about 4 minutes on one side, the turn over and grill for another 4 minutes, or until cooked through. Chicken should be charred but not burned.

17. Remove *Soft Baked Pita* from oven.

18. Peel and slice onion. Chop lettuce. Seed and chop tomato.

19. Spread pita with chilled *Tzatziki*. Add onion, lettuce and tomato over entire pita. Place chicken down center of pita.

20. Wrap up pita and serve immediately.

Gyro + Avocado Tzatziki

Prep Time: 5 minutes

Cook Time: 15 minutes

Servings: 1

INGREDIENTS

Soft Baked Pita

Quick Gyro Meat

4 oz ground lamb

4 oz ground beef

1/2 small onion

1 garlic clove

1/2 teaspoon dried marjoram

1/2 teaspoon dried oregano

1/2 teaspoon dried rosemary (ground or minced)

1/2 teaspoon ground black pepper

1/2 teaspoon sea salt

1 small rib romaine lettuce

1/2 tomato

1/2 small red onion

Avocado Tzatziki

1/2 small cucumber

1/2 avocado

1 teaspoon lemon juice

1 garlic clove

Pinch sea salt

1/2 teaspoon apple cider vinegar (optional)

2 mint leaves (optional)

INSTRUCTIONS

1. Preheat oven to 350 degrees F. Cover sheet pan with parchment paper or baking mat. Heat small pot over low heat. Line small loaf pan with parchment or aluminum foil.

2. Prepare *Soft Baked Pita* and place in oven.

3. For *Quick Gyro Meat*, peel onion and garlic while pita bakes. Add onion to food processor or bullet blender and process 10 - 15 seconds. Turn onion out onto cheesecloth or paper towels. Squeeze or compress onions to remove as much liquid as possible.

4. Add drained onions back to processor with lamb, beef, garlic, herbs, salt and pepper. Process until mixture is smooth. You may need to scrape down sides of bowl.

5. Spread meat mixture into bottom of prepared loaf pan and smooth top. Place in oven and bake for 10 minutes.

6. For *Avocado Tzatziki*, peel, seed and shred or grate cucumber. Peel and mince garlic. Mince mint. Slice avocado in half scoop flesh from one half into small mixing bowl. Add cucumber, garlic, lemon juice, salt, vinegar and mint (optional). Mix well, then place in refrigerator.

7. Heat medium skillet over medium-high heat and lightly coat with coconut oil.

8. Carefully remove loaf pan and release *Quick Gyro Meat*. Peel away parchment or aluminum and use tongs and sharp knife to cut lengthwise into 1/4 inch thick slices.

9. Add meat sliced to hot oiled skillet in single layer and sear about 5 minutes, until browned and cooked through. Turn over once while cooking. Meat should be charred but not burned.

10. Remove *Soft Baked Pita* from oven and let cool about 2 minutes.

11. Peel and slice red onion. Chop lettuce. Seed and chop tomato.

12. Spread pita with *Avocado Tzatziki*. Place meat down center of pita. Add lettuce, red onions and tomatoes over meat.

13. Wrap up pita and serve immediately.

Meatball Sub

Prep Time: 5 minutes

Cook Time: 20 minutes

Servings: 4

INGREDIENTS

Long Roll

Meatballs

1 lb ground meat (beef, pork, chicken, turkey, bison, or any combination)

3/4 cup almond flour

1 egg

1 garlic clove

1/2 small onion

1 teaspoon dried parsley

1 teaspoon dried oregano

1/2 teaspoon ground black pepper

1/2 teaspoon sea salt

1 tablespoon coconut oil

Tomato Sauce

1 can (8 oz) organic tomato sauce

1/4 cup water

1/2 teaspoon dried oregano

1/2 teaspoon dried basil

1/2 teaspoon ground black pepper

DIRECTIONS

1. Preheat oven to 350 degrees F. Line sheet pan with parchment paper, or lightly coat with coconut oil. Or lightly coat 6 mini loaf pans with coconut oil.

2. Prepare *Long Rolls* and place in oven.

3. While bread bakes, heat large pan over medium heat and add 1 tablespoon coconut oil.

4. For *Meatballs*, peel onion and garlic and add to food processor or blender. Pulse until finely processed, but before paste forms. Or finely mince.

5. Beat egg in large bowl. Add ground meat, almond flour, spices and salt. Mix well with hands or large wooden spoon.

6. Form 24 meatballs with scoop or tablespoon, then roll in hands. Add to hot pan and brown for 10 minutes. Turn with spatula or tongs to cook on all sides.

7. Add all *Tomato Sauce* ingredients to small pot and heat over low heat. Stir and simmer, until *Meatballs* in pan are browned.

8. Add *Meatballs* to simmering *Tomato Sauce* and increase heat to medium. Simmer another 5 minutes.

9. Remove *Long Rolls* from oven and let cool about 2 minutes.

10. Slice roll along side or split through top. Use slotted spoon to fill each roll with 6 meatballs.

11. Serve hot.

Cheese Steak Sandwich

Prep Time: 10 minutes*

Cook Time: 15 minutes

Servings: 4

INGREDIENTS

Long Roll

Almond Cheese

1 cup soaked skinless almonds*

1 tablespoons lemon juice

1 tablespoon apple cider vinegar

1 garlic clove

1/4 teaspoon ground black pepper

1/4 teaspoon paprika

1/2 teaspoon sea salt

1/4 cup water or 2 tablespoons coconut oil

Filling

1 lb beef steak

1 small onion

1 small bell pepper

1/2 teaspoon ground black pepper

1/2 teaspoon Sea salt

INSTRUCTIONS

1. *Soak almonds in enough water to cover overnight. Drain and rinse.

2. Preheat oven to 350 degrees F. Line sheet pan with parchment paper, or lightly coat with coconut oil. Or lightly coat 6 mini loaf pans with coconut oil.

3. Prepare *Long Rolls* and place in oven.

4. While bread bakes, heat medium skillet over medium-high heat.

5. Peel onion. Stem, vein and seed pepper. Thinly slice steak, onion and pepper.

6. Add steak to hot skillet and sauté about 1 minute. Add veggies, salt and pepper. Sauté about 5 minutes, until meat is cooked and veggies are soft and caramelized. Remove from heat.

7. Remove *Long Rolls* from oven and let cool about 2 minutes.

8. Add all *Almond Cheese* ingredients to food processor or bullet blender and process until smooth. Add 1 tablespoon water or coconut oil at a time to reach preferred consistency.

9. Slice roll along side or split through top and spread on *Almond Cheese*. Then layer on meat and veggies.

10. Serve immediately.

Veggie Burger

Prep Time: 5 minutes

Cook Time: 20 minutes

Servings: 4

INGREDIENTS

Soft Burger Bun

Veggie Burger

2 eggs

1/2 head cauliflower

2 medium carrots

1 small white onion

1 cup walnuts (1/2 cup ground)

1/4 cup almond flour

2 tablespoons tapioca flour

2 tablespoons ground chia seed (or flax meal)

2 cloves garlic

1 teaspoon paprika

1 teaspoon ground black pepper

1 teaspoon sea salt

Topping

1 avocado

1 heirloom tomato

1 white onion

2 ribs romaine lettuce (or preferred lettuce)

INSTRUCTIONS

1. Preheat oven to 350 degrees F. Line sheet pan with parchment paper, or lightly coat with coconut oil. Or lightly coat 6 mini round cake pans with coconut oil.

2. Prepare *Soft Burger Buns* and place in oven.

3. While bread bakes, line dish with parchment paper.

4. Add walnuts and almond four to food processor or bullet blender. Process until finely ground. Add to medium mixing bowl.

5. Peel small onion and garlic. Add to processor or blender with cauliflower and carrots. Process until finely ground. Add eggs, tapioca and chia. Process until mixture becomes thickened and has batter-like consistency.

6. Add veggie mixture and spices to mixing bowl. Mix all ingredients together with hands or wooden spoon until fully combined and uniform.

7. Form veggie mixture into 4 patties and place on parchment lined dish. Place in freezer for 10 minutes.

8. Heat medium skillet over medium-high heat and add 1 tablespoon coconut oil.

9. Peel onion. Make 4 thick slices, keeping full ring intact. Using spatula, place full rings into hot oiled pan. Sear 1 minute on each side. Set aside on paper towel to drain.

10. Reduce heat to medium and coat pan with coconut oil.

11. Remove veggie patties from freezer and place in hot oiled pan. Cook 5 minutes, then carefully flip with spatula and cook another 5 minutes.

12. Remove *Soft Burger Bun* from oven and let cool about 5 minutes.

13. Cut lettuce ribs in half. Cut tomato into 4 thick slices. Slice avocado in half, pit and slice flesh in peel.

14. Slice bun in half and place lettuce on bottom bun, followed by tomato slice. Add burger patty, then grilled onion ring. Finish with a few slices of avocado and top bun.

15. Serve immediately.

Crisp Spinach Salad

Prep Time: 15 minutes

Cook Time: 15 minutes

Servings: 2

INGREDIENTS

Spinach Salad

4 cups spinach

2 eggs

8 slices nitrate-free bacon

1 avocado

1 small onion

1/4 cup almond flour

1/2 teaspoon ground black pepper

1/4 teaspoon paprika

1/4 teaspoon sea salt

Bacon Vinaigrette

Bacon drippings

2 tablespoons coconut oil

2 tablespoons apple cider vinegar

1 teaspoon sweetener*

2 teaspoons organic mustard

1/4 teaspoon ground black pepper

INSTRUCTIONS

1. Bring small pot of lightly salted water to boil. Heat medium skillet over medium-high heat.

2. Gently add eggs to boiling water with tongs and boil about 7 - 10 minutes. Then remove and rinse under cold water. Crack shells and remove whole egg. Set aside.

3. While eggs cook, chop bacon and add to hot pan. Sauté about 5 - 8 minutes, until crisp and cooked through. Remove bacon and drain on paper towel. Reserve bacon drippings. Add drippings to small bowl once cooled slightly.

4. Lightly coat hot pan with coconut oil.

5. Add almond flour and spiced to small mixing bowl. Peel onion and cut in half. Cut onion into half-moon slices. Toss with almond flour until well coated.

6. Add coated onions to hot oiled pan. Let crisp about 1 - 2 minutes, then turn and continue cooking another minute, until fully crisp. Remove onion crisps and set aside on paper towel to drain.

7. Rinse, dry and plate spinach. Slice avocado in half, pit, and slice in peel. Slice eggs.

8. Add bacon pieces, avocado slices, sliced eggs and onion crisp to salads.

9. Add *Bacon Vinaigrette* ingredients to small bowl with reserved bacon grease and whisk well. Pour over salads.

10. Serve immediately.

*stevia raw honey or agave nectar

Egg Salad Sandwich

Prep Time: 5 minutes

Cook Time: 15 minutes

Servings: 2

INGREDIENTS

Sandwich Bread

Avocado Egg Salad

8 eggs

1 avocado

1/4 cup dill pickle relish

3 tablespoons organic mustard

2 teaspoons paprika

1/2 teaspoon ground black pepper

1/4 teaspoon sea salt

INSTRUCTIONS

1. Preheat oven to 350 degrees F. Lightly coat 6 mini round cake pans or medium loaf pan with coconut oil. Bring medium pot of lightly salted water to a boil.
2. Prepare *Sandwich Bread* and place in oven.
3. While bread bakes, gently add eggs to hot water with tongs and cook about 8 - 10 minutes.
4. Drain eggs in colander and run under cold water to cool.
5. While eggs cool, slice and pit avocado. Scoop flesh into medium mixing bowl. Add relish, mustard, salt and spices.

6. Crack eggs shells and peel. Add boiled eggs to medium mixing bowl.

7. Using a fork, mash ingredients together until smooth mixture with soft chunks forms.

8. Remove *Sandwich Bread* from oven and let cool about 5 minutes.

9. Slice bread and fill with *Avocado Egg Salad*.

10. Serve immediately. Or refrigerate about 20 minutes and serve chilled.

Kelp Noodle Salad

Prep Time: 5 minutes

Cook Time: 5 minutes

Servings: 2

INGREDIENTS

1 package (12 oz) kelp noodles

1/2 lemon

1 small cucumber

1 small red bell pepper

1 large carrot

Small bunch cilantro

2 large basil leaves

Orange Avocado Dressing

1 avocado

1 large orange

1/2 lemon

5 large basil leaves

1/4 teaspoon ground black pepper

1/4 teaspoon cayenne pepper or red pepper flake (optional)

Large bunch cilantro

INSTRUCTIONS

1. Rinse and drain kelp noodles. Add to medium bowl and soak 5
   minutes in warm water and juice of 1/2 lemon. Or bring medium

pot of water with juice of 1/2 lemon to a boil and cook kelp noodles for 5 minutes, if softer texture preferred.

2. Peel, seed and cut cucumber in half width-wise. Cut bell pepper in half, then remove stem, seeds and veins. Use vegetable peeler or grater to make long, thin slices of carrot. Thinly slice cucumber and bell pepper lengthwise.

3. Add veggies and drained kelp noodles to medium mixing bowl.

4. For *Orange Avocado Dressing*, add basil and cilantro leaves to food processor or bullet blender with juice of orange and process to break down leaves. Slice avocado in half and remove pit. Scoop flesh into processor with juice of 1/2 lemon, black pepper and hot pepper (optional). Process until thick and until creamy.

5. Pour *Orange Avocado Dressing* over sliced veggies and kelp noodles. Toss to coat.

6. Serve immediately. Or refrigerate for 20 minutes and serve chilled.

Dinner Recipes

Chicken Satay

Natural Orange Chicken

Cashew Chicken

Spicy Hunan Beef and Broccoli

Meaty Texas Chili

Spicy Meatball Marinara

Highland Sheppard's Pie

Black Pepper Stew

Nuts & Turkey Burgers

Chicken Bruschetta

Herb Roasted Pork Tenderloin

Ground Beef Stuffed Peppers

Stuffed Cabbage in Tomato Sauce

Slow Cooker Beef Pot Roast

Slow Cooker Beef Burgundy

Spicy Thai Soup

Natural Sweet Potato & Bacon Soup

Parchment Baked Salmon

Chicken Fries with Garlic Aioli

Ethiopian Beef Stew

Veggie Musakhan

Braised Lamb in Tomato Sauce

Garlic Sesame Chicken

Stewed Chicken and Dumplings

All-Natural Oven-Fried Chicken

Southern Liver and Onions

Spicy Oregano Cubes

French Country Coq Au Vin

Uptown Clam Chowder

Holiday Baked Ham

Chicken Satay

Prep Time: 10 minutes*

Cook Time: 25 minutes

Servings: 4

INGREDIENTS

16 oz (1 lb) boneless skinless chicken

12 wooden skewers (soaked in water for 1 hour)

Marinade

1 tablespoon pure fish sauce (or liquid aminos or coconut Aminos)

2 inch piece fresh ginger rot

1 garlic clove

Satay Sauce

13 oz (1 can) full-fat coconut milk

1/2 cup crunchy almond butter

1 tablespoon raw honey or agave nectar

1 tablespoon pure fish sauce (or tamari or coconut aminos)

1 teaspoon apple cider vinegar (or liquid aminos or coconut vinegar)

4 shallots

2 garlic cloves

2 inch piece fresh ginger root

2 small red chili peppers

1 1/2 tablespoons lime juice

Coconut oil (for cooking)

INSTRUCTIONS

1. *Cut chicken into 1 inch strips. For *Marinade*, peel and mince garlic and ginger. Add to medium mixing bowl with fish sauce and whisk. Add chicken and toss with until coated. Cover and set aside to marinate for 1 hour.

2. *Soak wooden skewers in water in shallow dish for 1 hour.

3. Heat medium pan or wok over medium heat and add 1 tablespoon coconut oil.

4. For *Satay Sauce*, peel and mince shallots, garlic and ginger. Slice peppers. Add to hot pan and sauté until softened, about 5 - 8 minutes.

5. Reduce heat to low. Add almond butter, coconut milk, honey, fish sauce, vinegar and lime juice. Whisk until blended. Gently simmer for 10 minutes. Remove from heat, but keep warm.

6. Preheat outdoor grill or griddle pan over medium-high heat. Lightly coat with coconut oil.

7. Pierce marinated chicken strips with soaked skewers. Pour some *Satay Sauce* over chicken and brush lightly with marinade brush to coat. Transfer remaining *Satay Sauce* to serving dish.

8. Grill chicken on preheated grill until just cooked through, about 3 minutes per side. Turn over skewers halfway through cooking. Do not overcook.

9. Remove skewers from heat and transfer to serving dish. Serve with *Satay Sauce*.

Natural Orange Chicken

Prep Time: 10 minutes

Cook Time: 10 minutes

Servings: 2

INGREDIENTS

12 oz (3/4 lb) boneless skinless chicken

1/2 cup almond flour

1 teaspoon flax meal

1 cage-free egg

1 green onion (scallion)

1/4 teaspoon cayenne pepper

1/2 teaspoon paprika

1/2 teaspoon ground black pepper

1/2 teaspoon Celtic sea salt

Coconut oil (for cooking)

Water

Orange Sauce

3 oranges (or tangerines or Clementines)

2 tablespoons raw honey (or agave)

1 tablespoon tamari (or liquid aminos or coconut aminos)

1 small garlic clove

1/2 inch piece fresh ginger

1/4 teaspoon ground black pepper

Water

INSTRUCTIONS

11. For *Orange Sauce*, zest 2 oranges, *then* juice all oranges into small pot. Peel and mince garlic and ginger. Add to pot with honey, tamari and pepper. Add 1/2 cup water.

12. Heat small pot over medium heat and bring to simmer. Simmer until *Orange Sauce* is reduced by half, about 5 minutes. Stir frequently. Remove from heat and set aside.

13. Heat medium pan over medium-high heat. Lightly coat pan with coconut oil.

14. In a shallow dish, blend almond meal, flax meal, salt and spices.

15. Whisk egg and 1 teaspoon water in separate shallow dish.

16. Cut chicken into 1 inch pieces. Dip chicken into egg wash, then dredge in seasoned almond meal.

17. Carefully place coated chicken pieces into hot oil and fry about 2 - 3 minutes, until golden brown and cooked through. Turn with tongs halfway through cooking.

18. Drain cooked chicken on paper towel, then transfer to medium mixing bowl. Pour *Orange Sauce* over chicken and toss to coat. Transfer to serving dish.

19. Slice scallions and sprinkle over dish. Serve hot.

Cashew Chicken

Prep Time: 5 minutes

Cook Time: 10 minutes

Servings: 2

INGREDIENTS

12 oz (3/4 lb) boneless skinless chicken

1/2 cup raw cashews

1/2 small onion (white or yellow)

1/2 red bell pepper

1/2 green bell pepper

1 small celery stalk

2 tablespoons tamari (or coconut aminos or apple cider vinegar)

1 teaspoon raw honey (or agave or date butter)

1 garlic clove

1/2 inch piece fresh ginger

1/4 teaspoon ground black pepper

1/2 teaspoon Celtic sea salt

Bacon fat or coconut oil (for cooking)

INSTRUCTIONS

1. Heat large pan or wok over medium heat. Lightly coat with bacon fat or coconut oil.

2. Peel and mince garlic and ginger. Remove seeds, stems and veins from peppers, then roughly chop. Dice carrot. Slice celery.

3. Roughly chop chicken and season with salt and pepper.

4. Add garlic and ginger to hot oiled pan or wok. Sauté about 1 minute, until fragrant. Add seasoned chicken add sauté until browned, about 2 minutes. Transfer chicken to small bowl and set aside.

5. Add veggies to hot oiled pan. Sauté until tender and lightly browned, about 2 minutes. Add tamari, honey and cashews. Sauté until veggies are just cooked, but still crisp.

6. Add chicken back to pan and heat until just cooked through, about 2 minutes.

7. Transfer to serving dish and serve hot.

Spicy Hunan Beef and Broccoli

Prep Time: 20 minutes

Cook Time: 10 minutes

Servings: 2

INGREDIENTS

12 oz (3/4 lb) beef sirloin

1/2 head broccoli

2 carrots

1 tablespoon tamari (or coconut aminos)

1 tablespoon dry sherry (or pure fish sauce or apple cider vinegar)

1 garlic clove

1/2 inch piece fresh ginger

1/2 teaspoon sesame seeds (optional)

Coconut oil (for cooking)

Sauce

1 tablespoon Asian chili paste

3 teaspoons tamari (or coconut aminos)

3 teaspoons chicken broth (or beef broth)

3 teaspoons dry sherry (or pure fish sauce or apple cider vinegar)

1 teaspoon raw honey (or agave)

1/2 teaspoon arrowroot flour

1/2 teaspoon sesame oil

2 garlic cloves

1/4 teaspoon fresh ground black pepper

INSTRUCTIONS

1. Cut beef against the grain into thin slices. Add to small mixing with tamari and sherry. And toss to coat. Set aside to marinate for 20 minutes.

2. For Sauce, peel and mince garlic. Add to small mixing bowl with chili paste, tamari, broth, sherry, honey, arrowroot, sesame oil and pepper. Mix to combine. Set aside.

3. Roughly chop broccoli into pieces. Slice carrots diagonally. Peel and mince garlic and ginger. Set aside.

4. Heat medium pan or wok over medium heat. Add 1 tablespoon coconut oil to hot pan.

5. Add marinated beef to hot pan in single layer. Let sear 1 minute on each side, undisturbed. Transfer to medium dish and set aside.

6. Add 1 tablespoon coconut oil to hot pan. Add garlic and ginger and sauté about 1 minute. Add broccoli and carrots. Sauté until lightly browned and softened, about 3 - 4 minutes. Stir frequently.

7. Add beef back to pan with *Sauce* and sesame seeds. Sauté until veggies are tender and beef is cooked through, about 2 minutes.

8. Transfer to serving dish and serve hot.

Meaty Texas Chili

Prep Time: 5 minutes

Cook Time: 40 minutes

Servings: 4

INGREDIENTS

16 oz (1 lb) lean grass-fed ground beef (or elk, bison, turkey or chicken)

15 oz (1 can) organic tomato sauce

29 oz (2 cans) organic diced tomatoes

1 cup water

1 cup cashews

1 small onion

1 bell pepper

2 cloves garlic

2 tablespoons chili powder

1 1/2 tablespoons smoked paprika (or paprika)

1 tablespoon ground cumin

1 teaspoon Mexican oregano (or dried oregano)

1 teaspoon ground black pepper

1/2 teaspoon cayenne pepper

1 teaspoon Celtic sea salt

1 tablespoon coconut oil

INSTRUCTIONS

7. Heat medium pot over medium-high heat. Add 1 tablespoon coconut oil to hot pan.

8. Peel onion and garlic. Remove stems, seeds and veins from bell pepper. Roughly chop and add to food processor or high-speed blender. Pulse until finely minced.

9. Add minced veggies to hot skillet and sauté for about 1 minute. Add ground beef and spices. Brown beef for about 5 minutes. Stir with whisk to break up meat well, or wooden spoon to keep beef chunkier.

10. Add whole cans of diced tomatoes and tomato sauce, and water. Stir to combine.

11. Bring to a simmer, then reduce heat to medium and cover pot loosely with lid to prevent splatter. Simmer about 30 minutes. Stir occasionally.

12. Remove from heat and transfer to serving dish. Use large serving spoon or ladle to serve hot.

Spicy Meatball Marinara

Prep Time: 5 minutes

Cook Time: 20 minutes

Servings: 4

INGREDIENTS

Meatballs

16 oz (1 lb) lean ground meat (beef, pork, chicken, turkey, bison, or any combination)

3/4 cup almond flour

1 cage-free egg

1/2 small onion (white, yellow or red)

1/2 teaspoon garlic powder

1/2 teaspoon cayenne pepper

1 teaspoon dried parsley

1 teaspoon dried oregano

1 teaspoon paprika

1 teaspoon red pepper flakes

1 teaspoon ground black pepper

1 teaspoon Celtic sea salt

1 tablespoon coconut oil

1 sprig fresh basil (for garnish, optional)

Tomato Sauce

14.5 oz (1 can) organic diced tomatoes

8 oz (1 can) organic tomato sauce

1 garlic clove

1/2 teaspoon dried oregano

1/2 teaspoon dried basil

1/2 teaspoon red pepper flakes

1/2 teaspoon ground black pepper

1 teaspoon coconut oil

INSTRUCTIONS

1. Heat large pan over medium heat. Add 1 tablespoon coconut oil to hot pan. Heat medium saucepan over medium heat. Add 1 teaspoon coconut oil.

2. For *Tomato Sauce*, peel garlic and mince. Add to medium saucepan and sauté until just golden, about 30 seconds. Add diced tomatoes, tomato sauce, salt and spices. Simmer about 5 - 10 minutes, stirring occasionally.

3. For *Meatballs*, peel onion process in food processor or high-speed blender, or finely grate.

4. Add to large mixing bowl. Add egg, ground meat, almond flour, spices and salt. Mix well with hands or large wooden spoon.

5. Form 24 meatballs with scoop or tablespoon, then roll in hands. Add meatballs to hot large pan and brown for 10 minutes. Turn with spatula or tongs to cook on all sides.

6. Add *Meatballs* to *Tomato Sauce* and simmer another 5 minutes.

7. Transfer *Meatballs* to serving dish. Top with simmering *Tomato Sauce*. Garnish with fresh basil (optional).

8. Serve hot.

Highland Sheppard's Pie

Prep Time: 20 minutes

Cook Time: 60 minutes

Servings: 4

INGREDIENTS

Meat Filling

24 oz (1 1/2 lbs) grass-fed ground lamb (or beef, bison, elk, etc.)

1 cup chicken broth or stock (or beef brother or stock, or red wine)

1 large onion (yellow or white)

2 carrots

6 - 10 asparagus stalks (about 1/2 cup chopped)

1/2 sweet potato (about 1/2 cup diced)

2 garlic cloves

1 tablespoon organic tomato paste

1 teaspoon tamari (or coconut aminos)

2 tablespoons tapioca flour (or arrow root powder)

1 sprig fresh rosemary

1 sprig fresh thyme

1/2 teaspoon ground black pepper (or ground white pepper)

1 teaspoon Celtic sea salt

Bacon fat or coconut oil (for cooking)

Parsnip Topping

4 medium parsnips

1/2 medium onion (yellow or white)

2 tablespoons cacao butter (or coconut oil)

2 cups water

3/4 teaspoon Celtic sea salt

1/2 ground white pepper (or ground black pepper) (optional)

INSTRUCTIONS

8. Heat medium pot over medium heat. Add 2 tablespoons bacon fat or coconut oil to hot pot.

9. For *Meat Filling*, peel and mince garlic. Peel and chop onion. Dice carrots and sweet potato. Chop asparagus. Add to hot oiled pot and sauté about 5 minutes.

10. Add lamb, salt and spices to veggies. Brown lamb and sauté another 5 minutes. Whisk in tapioca flour and cook another minute.

11. Remove rosemary and thymes leaves from stems and add to pot with stock, tomato paste and tamari. Let simmer and thicken about 12 minutes.

12. Preheat oven to 400 degrees F. Heat large pan with lid over medium heat. Add butter or oil to hot pan.

13. For *Parsnip Topping*, peel and mince or finely grate onion. Add to hot pan and sauté until translucent and aromatic, about 2 minutes.

14. Peel and slice or chop parsnips. Add to onions with water. Increase heat to high and bring to a simmer. Cover pan loosely with lid. Cook parsnips partially covered until softened and most of the water has evaporated, about 10 minutes.

15. Pour parsnips and onions into food processor or high-speed blender. Process until thick, smooth mixture forms. Add enough water to reach desired consistency. Set aside.

16. Transfer *Meat Filling* to baking or casserole dish. Top with *Parsnip Topping*. Smooth over or create design with offset spatula or back of spoon.

17. Bake about 25 minutes, until *Parsnip Topping* is golden.

18. Remove from oven and let cool at least 10 minutes. Serve warm.

Black Pepper Stew

Prep time: 15 minutes

Cook time: 3 hr 45 minutes

Serves: 6

INGREDIENTS

1 ½ lbs beef stew meat

1 onion

1 (14.5 oz) can no-salt added stewed tomatoes, undrained

¼ tsp Celtic sea salt

½ tsp ground black pepper

1 dried bay leaf

2 cups water

3 tbsp arrowroot powder

12 small sweet potatoes cut in half

30 baby-cut carrots

INSTRUCTIONS

1. Heat oven to 325 degrees. In a bowl, mix arrowroot in water and stir to a paste (if you're not using arrowroot, use 1 cup water instead). Cut the onion into 8 wedges and cut potatoes in half.

2. In ovenproof Dutch oven, mix beef, onion, tomatoes, Celtic sea salt, ground black pepper and bay leaf. Mix arrowroot-thickened water (or 1 cup water) into Dutch oven.

3. Cover and bake for 2 hours, stirring one time.

4. Stir in the potatoes and carrots. Cover and bake until beef and vegetables are tender, about 1 hr 45 min. Remove bay leaf and serve immediately, or chill 20 minutes and then serve.

Nuts & Turkey Burgers

Prep time: 10 minutes

Cook time: 6-12 minutes

Servings: 4

INGREDIENTS

16 oz ground turkey

1 cup walnuts

2 cloves garlic

1 onion

¼ tsp chipotle chili pepper powder

¼ tbsp smoked paprika

¼ tsp ground black pepper

INSTRUCTIONS

1. Chop walnuts into smaller pieces, about ⅛" cubes. Mince garlic and chop onion into small pieces, about ¼" pieces.
2. Combine the above with ground turkey and add chipotle chili pepper powder, smoked paprika and ground black pepper. Knead it all together and separate into four patties.
3. Cook on the grill on high heat, flipping occasionally, until desired done-ness.

Chicken Bruschetta

Prep time: 10 minutes

Cook time: 10 minutes

Serves: 4

INGREDIENTS

4 grass-fed chicken breasts

2 tomatoes

4 olives

2 onions

¼ tsp ground black pepper

1 cup roasted red pepper

3 tbsp extra virgin olive oil

INSTRUCTIONS

1. Dice the tomatoes, chop the olives and onions, and combine them with ground black pepper and 2 tbsp olive oil in a bowl and mix well into a bruschetta. Puree the roasted red pepper in a blender and set aside.

2. Combine the chicken with 1 tbsp extra virgin olive oil and cook in a pan over medium-high heat for 4 minutes, turn once, and cook another 4-6 minutes, removing from heat while still tender.

3. Place one piece of chicken on each plate and pour the roasted red pepper over each, adding bruschetta over the top. Garnish with basil and serve.

Herb Roasted Pork Tenderloin

Prep Time: 10 minutes*

Cook Time: 15 minutes

Servings: 4

INGREDIENTS

1 pork tenderloin

1 teaspoon dried rosemary

1 teaspoon dried thyme

1 teaspoon dried oregano

1 teaspoon dried basil

1 teaspoon dried marjoram (optional)

1/2 teaspoon ground black pepper

1 teaspoon Celtic sea salt

Apricot Sauce

1 cup dried apricots

2/3 cup water

1 teaspoon apple cider vinegar (or dry white wine)

INSTRUCTIONS

1. Preheat oven to 425 degrees F. Heat small pan over medium heat.

2. Rub tenderloin with salt and spices, then press into meat so it adheres. Place on sheet pan, or wire rack over sheet pan.

3. Roast for 10 - 15 minutes, until just cooked through and no pink remains. Remove pork from oven and let rest 10 minutes.

4. For *Apricot Sauce*, add dried apricots, water and vinegar to food processor or high-speed blender. Process until smooth, about 1 - 2 minutes.

5. Add *Apricot Sauce* to hot pan and reduce until slightly thickened. Stir well and do not let burn. Remove from heat.

6. Slice pork and transfer to serving dish. Top pork with *Apricot Sauce* and serve warm.

Ground Beef Stuffed Peppers

Prep Time: 10 minutes

Cook Time: 50 minutes

Servings: 4

INGREDIENTS

4 bell peppers

16 oz (1 lb) ground meat (beef, pork, chicken, turkey, etc.)

1/2 head cauliflower (1 cup riced)

1/2 cup roasted red peppers

1/4 cup sundried tomatoes

1/4 cup pecans

1/2 small onion (white, yellow or red)

2 tablespoons coconut oil

2 garlic cloves

Medium bunch fresh herbs (parsley, oregano, thyme, etc.)

1/4 teaspoon red pepper flakes

1 teaspoon ground white pepper (or black pepper)

1 teaspoon Celtic sea salt

Water

INSTRUCTIONS

1. Preheat oven to 350 degrees F.
2. Cut tops off peppers, then remove stems from tops and seeds and veins from bottoms of peppers. Leave bottoms of peppers hollow

but do not pierce. Place in baking dish just large enough to fit peppers snuggly. Set aside.

3. Peel onion and garlic. Roughly chop onions, garlic and cauliflower. Add to food processor or high-speed blender with pecans. Pulse about 15 seconds.

4. Add tops of peppers, roasted red peppers, sundried tomatoes, ground meat, salt, pepper, and fresh herbs to processor. Process until coarsely ground, about 1 - 2 minutes.

5. Use large spoon to stuff peppers with mixture. Add 1/2 cup water to bottom of baking dish. Cover peppers with aluminum foil.

6. Bake 30 minutes. Carefully remove foil and continue baking uncovered 10 - 20 minutes, until stuffing is golden brown and cooked through .

7. Carefully remove from oven and transfer peppers to serving dish. Serve hot.

Stuffed Cabbage in Tomato Sauce

Prep Time: 15 minutes

Cook Time: 60 minutes

Servings: 6

INGREDIENTS

1 large cabbage head

Filling

2 1/2 lbs ground beef

4 cage-free eggs

1/2 onion (yellow or white)

1/3 cup almond flour

1/2 cup cauliflower (riced or minced)

1/2 teaspoon dried thyme

1/2 teaspoon ground black pepper (or ground white pepper)

1 1/2 teaspoons Celtic sea salt

Tomato Sauce

2 cans (15 oz) organic tomato sauce

1/2 cup golden raisins

1/2 onion (yellow or white)

2 tablespoons raw honey (or agave or date butter)

2 tablespoons apple cider vinegar

1 1/2 teaspoons Celtic sea salt

1 teaspoon ground black pepper (or ground white pepper)

2 tablespoons bacon fat (or coconut oil or ghee)

INSTRUCTIONS

1. Preheat oven to 350 degrees F. Bring large pot of salted water to boil.

2. Carefully place cabbage head in boiling water for about 5 minutes. Use tongs to peel each layer of leaves from head as soon as they become tender. Set leaves aside on sheet pan to cool.

3. For *Tomato Sauce*, peel and mince onions. Add 1/2 of onions to medium mixing bowl. Add tomato sauce, honey, vinegar, raisins, salt and spices and mix to combine.

4. For *Filling*, add remaining onions to large mixing bowl. Mince or rice cauliflower and add to bowl with eggs, almond flour, salt, spices, and 1 cup *Tomato Sauce*. Mix well with hands or large wooden spoon.

5. Cut hard rib from bottom of each cooled cabbage leaf. Place 1/3 - 1/2 cup *Filling* near the bottom edge of cabbage leaf and roll into a neat package, tucking in sides as you roll. Repeat with remaining filling and cabbage.

6. Spread 1 cup *Tomato sauce* along bottom of deep, lidded baking dish. Place 1/2 the cabbage rolls in baking dish. Add 1/2 remaining sauce, the remaining cabbage rolls. Top with remaining sauce.

7. Tightly cover dish with lid and bake for 1 hour, until meat is cooked through and veggies are tender.

8. Transfer to serving dish and serve hot.

Slow Cooker Beef Pot Roast

Prep Time: 20 minutes

Cook Time: 6 hours

Servings: 8

INGREDIENTS

5 lb bone-in beef pot roast (or bone-in beef chuck)

2 1/2 cups chicken stock (or broth)

1 1/2 cups button mushrooms (about 1/2 pint)

3 carrots

2 celery stalks

1 onion (white or yellow)

2 garlic cloves

2 1/2 tablespoons tapioca flour (or arrowroot powder)

1 tablespoon organic tomato paste

2 sprigs fresh thyme

1 sprig fresh rosemary

1 - 2 tablespoons ground black pepper

1 - 2 tablespoons Celtic sea salt

1 tablespoon ghee (or cacao butter)

2 tablespoons coconut oil (for cooking)

INSTRUCTIONS

1. Heat large skillet over medium-high heat. Add coconut oil to hot pan.

2. Generously season beef on all sides with salt and pepper. Sprinkle 1 tablespoon tapioca or arrowroot over beef and pat to coat. Add to hot oiled pan and sear on all sides until browned, about 5 minutes per side. Set aside in baking dish to rest.

3. Slice mushrooms. Peel and chop onions. Peel and mince garlic.

4. Add ghee or butter and mushrooms to hot pan. Sauté about 2 minutes.

5. Add onions and sauté until translucent, about 5 minutes. Add garlic and sauté about 1 minute.

6. Stir in remaining 1 1/2 tablespoons tapioca or arrowroot and cook about 1 minute. Stir in tomato paste.

7. Slowly stir in chicken stock and bring to simmer, about 5 minutes. Remove from heat.

8. Roughly chop carrots and celery. Add to bottom of slow cooker. Place rested beef over veggies and pour in any juices from beef. Add rosemary and thyme. Add mushroom mixture over beef.

9. Cover slow cooker with lid. Turn on to high and cook 5 - 6 hours, until beef is fork tender.

10. Turn off slow cooker and carefully remove lid. Skim off any fat from surface and remove bones.

11. Transfer to serving dish and serve hot.

Slow Cooker Beef Burgundy

Prep Time: 30 minutes

Cook Time: 7 hours

Servings: 6

INGREDIENTS

3 lbs boneless stew beef

2 cups beef stock (or broth)

1 bottle (750 ml) organic dry red wine

1/2 cup organic sparkling apple cider (or cognac)

8 oz (1/2 lb) nitrate-free bacon

1 pint fresh mushrooms (about 2 cups)

4 large carrots

2 yellow onions

2 cups whole pearl onions (peeled)

2 garlic cloves

1 tablespoon organic tomato paste

3 tablespoons tapioca flour (arrowroot powder)

1/2 teaspoon dried thyme

1 teaspoon ground black pepper

2 teaspoons Celtic sea salt

2 tablespoons coconut oil (for cooking)

INSTRUCTIONS

1. Heat large skillet over medium-high heat. Add coconut oil to hot pan.

2. Cut beef into chunks than add to large mixing bowl. Season beef with salt and pepper, then add 2 tablespoons tapioca or arrowroot. Toss to coat.

3. Add seasoned beef to hot oiled pan in batches to brown, about 5 minutes per batch. Set aside in slow cooker.

4. Chop bacon and add to hot pan. Sauté until just crisp and fat renders out, about 5 - 8 minutes. Set aside in slow cooker.

5. Peel and chop yellow onions. Peel and mince garlic. Add to hot bacon grease and sauté about 5 minutes. Set aside in slow cooker.

6. Cut mushrooms in half. Add to hot pan with tomato paste, remaining tapioca or arrow root, thyme and apple cider. Stir to combine. Then add beef stock to deglaze pan. Bring to simmer, about 5 minutes.

7. Pour mushroom mixture into slow cooker. Add red wine and peeled pearl onions. Chop carrots and add to slow cooker. Stir to combine.

8. Cover slow cooker with lid. Turn on to low and cook 6 - 8 hours, until meat and veggies are tender.

9. Turn off slow cooker and carefully remove lid.

10. Transfer to serving dish and serve hot.

Spicy Thai Soup

Prep Time: 15 minutes

Cook Time: 1 hour

Servings: 4

INGREDIENTS

1 3/4 lbs boneless skinless chicken thighs

4 cups chicken broth (or stock)

1 can (14 oz) coconut milk (lite or full-fat)

1 1/2 cups white mushrooms

2 lemongrass stalks

1 small red onion

3 garlic cloves

3 inch piece ginger root

2 tablespoons pure fish sauce

1 1/2 teaspoons red curry paste

2 limes

1 jalapeño pepper

Small bunch cilantro

1 tablespoon coconut oil

Water

INSTRUCTIONS

1. Thinly slice bottom 2/3 of lemongrass. Peel chop garlic and ginger. Add to medium pot with chicken broth. Heat over medium-high-heat and bring to boil.

2. Reduce heat to low and simmer for 30 minutes. Strain liquid and reserve.

3. Heat pot over medium heat. Add coconut oil to hot pot.

4. Roughly chop chicken and add to hot oiled pot. Sauté and brown for 5 minutes. Quarter mushrooms and add to pot. Sauté for 5 minutes.

5. Stir in red curry paste, fish sauce, and juice of 1 lime. Add reserved chicken broth and coconut milk. Stir to combine and bring to a simmer.

6. Reduce heat to low and simmer 15 - 20 minutes. Skim off and discard any excess fat that rises to the top.

7. Peel and slice red onion. Add to pot and stir. Cook about 5 minutes, until onion softens.

8. Remove from heat. Roughly chop add 1/2 to pot and stir to combine.

9. Slice jalapeño into rings and cut lime into wedges.

10. Transfer to serving dish. Sprinkle remaining cilantro and jalapeño slices over dish.

11. Serve hot with lime wedges.

Natural Sweet Potato & Bacon Soup

Prep Time: 20 minutes

Cook Time: 1 hour 20 minutes

Servings: 4

INGREDIENTS

4 cups chicken broth (or veggie broth)

2 large sweet potatoes (yams)

8 oz (1/2 lb) nitrate free bacon

1 cup full-fat coconut milk

1/4 teaspoon cayenne pepper

1/2 teaspoon ground cinnamon

1/2 teaspoon dried thyme

1 teaspoon ground black pepper

Celtic sea salt, to taste

INSTRUCTIONS

1. Preheat oven to 400 degrees F. Line sheet pan with parchment or baking mat.

2. Cut sweet potatoes crosswise into thick slices and lay on prepared sheet pan. Sprinkle with salt and pepper, to taste.

3. Roast sweet potatoes for about 45 minutes, until golden brown and cooked through. Remove from oven and allow to cool slightly. Then remove skin from sweet potatoes.

4. Heat medium pot over medium-high heat.

5. Chop bacon and add to hot pot. Sauté bacon until crisp, about 7 - 8 minutes. Remove bacon and set aside.

6. Add bacon fat to food processor or high-speed blender with peeled sweet potatoes and broth. Process until puréed.

7. Or add peeled sweet potatoes and broth to pot and purée in with immersion blender.

8. Add spices and coconut milk and stir to combine. Reduce heat to medium and let simmer about 10 minutes.

9. Transfer to serving dish and sprinkle with crisp bacon. Serve hot.

Parchment Baked Salmon

Prep Time: 5 minutes

Cook Time: 20 minutes

Servings: 1

INGREDIENTS

8 oz salmon fillet (deboned, skin-on)

6 - 8 medium asparagus stalks

1/2 lemon

1 basil sprig

1 rosemary sprig

1 teaspoon coconut oil

Pinch black pepper

Pinch sea salt

Parchment paper

Kitchen twine

INSTRUCTIONS

1. Place large sheet pan on bottom rack of oven. Preheat oven to 400 degrees F. prepare parchment sheet.
2. Place salmon in middle of parchment sheet skin-side down and sprinkle with salt and pepper. Place asparagus stalks next to salmon. Cut lemon into thin slices and place over fish and asparagus. Rub herbs between palms, then lay basil and rosemary sprig over lemon slices. Drizzle 1 teaspoon coconut oil over salmon and asparagus.

3. Gather edges of parchment up over salmon and tie tightly with kitchen twine to form sealed pouch.

4. Place pouch directly on hot baking sheet in hot oven. Bake for 20 minutes.

5. Remove from oven and carefully transfer pouch to serving plate. Carefully open pouch to release steam.

6. Serve hot.

Chicken Fries with Garlic Aioli

Prep Time: 10 minutes

Cook Time: 15 minutes

Servings: 2

INGREDIENTS

8 oz boneless, skinless chicken breast

1 egg

1/2 cup almond meal

1 teaspoon flax meal (or ground chia seed)

1 teaspoon ground black pepper

1/2 teaspoon paprika

1/2 teaspoon onion powder

1/2 teaspoon garlic powder

1/2 teaspoon chili powder

1/2 teaspoon sea salt

Garlic Aioli

1/2 - 3/4 cup coconut oil

1 egg yolk

2 garlic cloves

1/2 small lemon

1/4 teaspoon ground white pepper (or black pepper)

1/4 teaspoon sea salt

3 tablespoons flavorful oil (black truffle, walnut, almond, sesame, etc.)

(optional)

INSTRUCTIONS

1. Heat large pan over medium-high heat and coat with coconut oil.

2. For *Garlic Aioli*, peel garlic and add to food processor or blender with egg yolk, juice of 1/2 lemon, salt and pepper. Process until smooth, scraping down sides of vessel.

3. While processor or blender is running, very slowly drizzle in enough coconut oil to create thick mayo-like mixture. Drizzle in flavorful oil as well will processor runs (optional). If mixture is runny, drizzle in more coconut oil while processor runs until thickened. Pour into serving dish and refrigerate.

4. Slice chicken into half width-wise, creating twice the fillets. Try to slice at thickest portion to keep all fillets equal thickness.

5. Slice chicken fillets into long, 1/2 inch wide strips. Place strips between two paper towels and press to absorb excess moisture.

6. In a shallow dish, blend almond meal, flax or chia meal, spices and salt.

7. Beat egg in small mixing bowl. Toss chicken strips in beaten egg to lightly coat, then dredge in seasoned almond meal.

8. Carefully place coated chicken strips into hot oil and fry about 2 - 3 minutes, until golden brown and cooked through. Turn with tongs half way through cooking.

9. Drain cooked chicken on paper towel, then transfer to serving dish.

10. Serve hot with *Garlic Aioli*.

Ethiopian Beef Stew

Prep Time: 30 minutes

Cook Time: 1 hour

Servings: 4

INGREDIENTS

24 oz (1 1/2 lb) stew beef

2 cups beef stock (or chicken or veggie stock)

2 tablespoons organic tomato paste

1/2 teaspoon raw honey (or agave or date butter)

1 small onion

2 garlic cloves

2 teaspoons Celtic sea salt

2 teaspoons *Spice Blend*

2 tablespoons ghee (or cacao butter or bacon fat)

3 tablespoons coconut oil (or bacon fat)

Spice Blend

1/8 teaspoon ground nutmeg

1/8 teaspoon ground allspice

1/8 teaspoon turmeric

1/4 teaspoon ground cumin

1/4 teaspoon ground cinnamon

1/4 teaspoon ground cloves

1/4 teaspoon garlic powder

1/2 teaspoon ground black pepper

1/2 teaspoon ground fenugreek

1/2 teaspoon ground ginger

1/2 teaspoon ground coriander

1/2 teaspoon cardamom seed (or 1/4 teaspoon ground cardamom)

1 teaspoon dried onion flakes (or 1/2 teaspoon onion powder)

1 tablespoon paprika

2 tablespoons red pepper flakes

INSTRUCTIONS

1. Heat medium pot over medium-high heat. Add Spice blend and toast until fragrant. Stir frequently and do not burn. Remove toasted *Spice Blend* and set aside.

2. Add ghee and coconut oil to hot pot.

3. Cut beef into 1 inch chunks. Set aside.

4. Peel onion and garlic. Mince garlic and dice onion. Add to hot oiled pot and sauté until caramelized, about 2 - 3 minutes.

5. Add tomato paste, 2 teaspoons *Spice Blend* and honey to pot. Stir and cook into thick paste, about 2 minutes. Stir in a few tablespoon of beef stock to loosen paste.

6. Add beef, remaining beef stock and salt to pot. Stir to combine. Reduce heat to medium-low and simmer until beef is tender and sauce thickens and reduces, about 1 hour. Stir occasionally.

7. Transfer to serving dish and serve room temperature.

Veggie Musakhan

Prep time: 4 minutes

Cook time: 8 minutes

Servings: 4

INGREDIENTS

4 pieces grass-fed chicken thighs

1 onion

2 cloves garlic

3/4 cup sliced carrots

2 handfuls Kale greens

2 tbsp chinese five spice

2 tbsp smoked paprika

2 tbsp chipotle chili pepper powder

1 tbsp olive oil

2 tsp lemon juice

1 tbsp coconut oil

INSTRUCTIONS

1. Mince garlic and chop onion to desired size (medium strips work best). Chop carrots to 1/4" thickness. De-rib the kale and chop it coarsely, wash it and allow water to remain on the leaves. Bring 4 cups of water to a light boil.

2. Heat 1 tbsp olive oil over medium heat in a large pan. Add carrot and onion and cook for 8 minutes, stirring occasionally.

3. Meanwhile, heat 1 tbsp coconut oil over medium heat in a separate pan. Add chicken and cook for 4 minutes. Season chicken with chinese five spice, chipotle chili pepper powder and smoked paprika and turn, adding more of each spice to the other side of the chicken, cooking for another 4 minutes or until cooked through.

4. Add kale to boiling water and boil until bright green, about 5 minutes. Remove from water and let sit while the vegetables and chicken continue cooking.

5. Add everything into the pan with the vegetables and add 2 tsp lemon juice. Add minced garlic and stir for 1 minute.

6. Serve immediately.

Braised Lamb in Tomato Sauce

Prep Time: 20 minutes

Cook Time: 9 hours

Servings: 4

INGREDIENTS

3 lbs bone-in lamb shank

1 can (15 oz) organic tomato sauce

1 can (15 oz) organic crushed tomatoes

1/4 cup red wine (or apple cider vinegar)

2 cups pearl onions (peeled)

2 garlic cloves

1 teaspoon dried oregano

1 teaspoon dried thyme

1 teaspoon paprika

1 teaspoon ground black pepper

2 teaspoons Celtic sea salt

1 tablespoon coconut oil (for cooking)

Chicken stock (or water)

INSTRUCTIONS

1. Heat medium skillet over medium-high heat. Add coconut oil to hot pan.
2. Add lamb to hot oiled pan and sear on all sides, about 3 - 4 minutes per side. Set aside in slow cooker.

3. Peel pearl onions. Peel and mince garlic. Add to hot oiled pan and sauté about 2 minutes.

4. Add tomatoes sauce, red wine or vinegar, salt and spices to pan. Stir to combine.

5. Add to slow cooker with crushed tomatoes enough chicken stock or water to cover lamb.

6. Cover slow cooker with lid. Turn on to medium and cook 4 - 5 hours, until meat is tender.

7. Turn off slow cooker and carefully remove lid.

8. Transfer to serving dish and serve hot.

Garlic Sesame Chicken

Prep Time: 10 minutes

Cook Time: 20 minutes

Servings: 2

INGREDIENTS

12 oz (3/4 lb) boneless skinless chicken

1/4 cup almond flour

1/4 cup arrowroot powder

1 large cage-free egg white

2 teaspoon sesame seeds

1/4 teaspoon cayenne pepper

1/2 teaspoon garlic powder

1/2 teaspoon ground black pepper

1/2 teaspoon Celtic sea salt

Coconut oil (for cooking)

Garlic Sauce

1/2 yellow onion

1/2 lemon

6 garlic cloves

1/4 inch piece fresh ginger

1/4 cup date butter (or raw honey or agave)

2 tablespoons pure fish sauce

2 tablespoons coconut aminos (or tamar or liquid aminos)

2 tablespoons tamari (or liquid aminos or coconut aminos)

1/4 teaspoon ground black pepper

Water

INSTRUCTIONS

1. For *Garlic Sauce*, peel onions, garlic and ginger. Roughly chop and add to food processor or high-speed blender. Add date butter, fish sauce, coconut aminos, tamari and black pepper. Process until smooth.

2. Add sesame seeds to small pot. Heat over medium heat and toast about 2 minutes. Stir constantly. Transfer to small bowl and set aside.

3. Pour *Garlic Sauce* into pot and cook until onions and date butter until caramelized and garlic is fragrant, about 5 minutes. Stir frequently.

4. Add enough water to create saucy consistency. Stir frequently and bring to simmer. Simmer until *Garlic Sauce* is reduced by half and browned, about 5 minutes. Remove from heat and set aside.

5. Heat medium pan over medium-high heat. Coat pan with about 1/4 inch coconut oil.

6. In a shallow dish, blend almond meal, arrowroot powder, salt and spices.

7. Beat egg whites in small mixing bowl with hand mixer or whisk until light and frothy, about 2 - 4 minutes.

8. Cut chicken into 1 inch pieces. Dip chicken in egg whites, then dredge in seasoned flour mixture.

9. Carefully place coated chicken pieces into hot oil and fry about 2 - 3 minutes, until golden brown and cooked through. Turn with tongs halfway through cooking.

10. Drain cooked chicken on paper towel, then transfer to medium mixing bowl. Pour *Garlic Sauce* and 1 teaspoon toasted sesame seeds over chicken and toss to coat. Transfer to serving dish.
11. Sprinkle remaining toasted sesame seeds over dish. Serve hot.

Stewed Chicken and Dumplings

Prep Time: 10 minutes

Cook Time: 1 hour 20 minutes

Servings: 4

INGREDIENTS

2 lb whole chicken (innards removed)

6 - 10 cups water

3 carrots

3 celery stalks

1 small white onion (or yellow onion)

4 bay leaves

1 1/2 tablespoons dried thyme (or 4 sprigs fresh thyme)

1/2 teaspoon dried oregano

1 teaspoon paprika

2 teaspoon ground black pepper

1 tablespoon Celtic sea salt

Dumplings

3 cups almond flour

1/2 cup arrowroot powder

2 cage-free egg

1/2 cup coconut oil, chilled (or coconut or cacao butter, room temperature)

1/2 teaspoon baking soda

1/4 teaspoon ground bay leaf

1 teaspoon dried thyme

1/2 teaspoon ground white pepper (or ground black pepper)

1 teaspoon Celtic sea salt

Nut milk (or chicken broth or stock)

INSTRUCTIONS

1. Heat large pot over medium-high heat. Place chicken breast-down in hot pot. Sear chicken and turn to brown and render out fat for about 15 minutes.

2. Chop carrots and celery. Peel onion and mince. Add to chicken with salt and spices. Sauté about 2 minutes.

3. Add enough water to pot to cover chicken. Increase heat to high and bring to a boil. Reduce heat to medium and simmer about 30 minutes. Place lid loosely over pot to prevent splatter, if necessary.

4. For *Dumplings*, sift almond flour and arrowroot into medium mixing bowl. Cut in solid oil or butter with fork until crumbly mixture forms. Add egg, salt and spices, baking soda, and enough nut milk or chicken broth from pot to bring together soft, slightly sticky dough.

5. Carefully remove chicken from pot with long utensil and set aside. Use utensils to remove skin from chicken. Carve chicken into desired pieces and place back in back.

6. Use spoon or scoop to gently drop dough into pot. Cover with well-fitting lid and let simmer about 15 - 20 minutes, until *Dumplings* and chicken are cooked through. Gently stir soup to periodically prevent *Dumplings* from sticking. Turn over any *Dumplings* that are not submerged.

7. Remove from heat and transfer to serving dish. Serve hot.

All-Natural Oven-Fried Chicken

Prep Time: 10 minutes

Cook Time: 60 minutes

Servings: 4

INGREDIENTS

32 oz (2 lb) bone-in, skinless chicken

3/4 cup fine almond flour

3/4 cup coarse almond meal (or almond flour)

2 cage free eggs

1/3 cup nut milk

1/2 teaspoon cayenne pepper

1 teaspoon ground black pepper

1 1/2 teaspoons paprika

1 1/2 tablespoons Celtic sea salt

Coconut oil (in spray bottle)

INSTRUCTIONS

1. Preheat oven to 350 degrees F. Fill spray bottle with warm coconut oil.

2. Line sheet pan with aluminum foil. Place metal cooling or baking rack over lined sheet pan. Generously spray metal rack with coconut oil to coat. Set second sheet pan aside.

3. Add almond meal and/or flour to small mixing bowl with 1 tablespoon salt and spices. Mix to combine with fork or whisk to break up clumps.

4. In shallow dish, beat eggs and nut milk until combined.

5. Use serving spoon or measuring cup to dust second sheet pan with layer of almond flour mixture onto. Sprinkle chicken with 1/2 tablespoon salt.

6. Dip and coat all chicken pieces in egg mixture then lay on second sheet pan, over layer of almond flour mixture. Use spoon or measuring cut to sprinkle almond flour mixture from mixing bowl over dipped chicken. Pat almond flour mixture into chicken on all sides until well coated.

7. Transfer coasted chicken to prepared wire rack. Generously spray coated chicken with coconut oil.

8. Bake 60 - 70 minutes, until coating is crisp and chicken is cooked through. Remove from oven and allow to cool at least 10 minutes. Then place crispy chicken on paper towels to drain, if desired.

9. Transfer to serving dish and serve immediately.

Southern Liver and Onions

Prep Time: 20 minutes*

Cook Time: 25 minutes

Servings: 4

INSTRUCTIONS

20 oz (1 1/4 lb) calves liver

2 onions (yellow or white)

4 slices nitrate-free bacon

1 lemon

2 tablespoons arrowroot powder

1/2 teaspoon Celtic sea salt

1/2 teaspoon cracked black pepper (or ground black pepper)

 Bacon fat or coconut oil (for cooking)

INSTRUCTIONS

10. *Remove thin outer membrane from liver and slice into 1/4 inch
    fillets. Add to glass container. Juice lemon into container and toss
    to coat. Cover well and refrigerate overnight.

11. Heat large cast-iron pan or skillet set over medium heat.

12. Cut bacon lengthwise into long, thin strips. Then cut in thirds
    crosswise and add to hot pan. Sauté bacon and let crisp, about 5
    minutes. Stir occasionally. Decrease heat to medium-low.

13. Peel and thinly slice onions. Add to bacon and sauté until
    caramelized, about 10 minutes. Stir occasionally. Remove
    caramelized onions and bacon from pan and set aside.

14. Drain liver fillets in colander in sink. Rinse under running water, then pat dry.
15. In shallow dish, add arrowroot powder, salt and pepper. Mix with fork to combine.
16. Dredge liver slices in arrowroot mixture and shake off excess. Place coated liver fillets on a plate and coat remaining liver fillets.
17. Add 2 tablespoons bacon fat or coconut oil to hot pan. Add single layer of coated liver to hot oiled pan and sear for 1 minute per side. Place liver on paper towel to drain. Repeat with remaining liver.
18. Transfer liver to serving dish. Top with caramelized onions and bacon. Serve immediately .

Spicy Oregano Cubes

Prep time: 1 hr 10 minutes

Cook time: 16-20 minutes

Serves: 4

INGREDIENTS

1 boneless leg of lamb

5 tbsp extra virgin olive oil

2 tsp dried oregano

1 tbsp fresh parsley

1 lemon

½ eggplant

4 small onions

2 tomatoes

5 fresh bay leaves

¼ tsp Celtic sea salt

¼ tsp ground black pepper

INSTRUCTIONS

1. Cube the lamb, chop the fresh parsley, juice the lemon, slice and quarter the eggplant into thick pieces, halve the onions and quarter the tomatoes.

2. Place lamb in a bowl. Mix olive oil, oregano, parsley, lemon juice and Celtic sea salt and ground black pepper. Pour this over the lamb and mix well. Cover and marinate for 1 hour.

3. Preheat the grill. Thread the marinated lamb, eggplant, onions, tomatoes and bay leaves in evenly on each of four skewers.

4. Place the kebabs on a grill inside a grill pan and brush them evenly with the leftover marinade until the marinade is all gone. Cook over medium heat turning once the kebabs once, for about 8-10 minutes on each side, basting them whenever enough juice collects in the bottom of the grill pan.

5. Serve immediately or chill 20 minutes and then serve.

French Country Coq Au Vin

Prep Time: 30 minutes

Cook Time: 7 hours

Servings: 6

1 (5 - 7 lb) stewing chicken (innards removed)

2 cups chicken stock (or broth)

2 bottles(750 ml) organic red wine

6 oz nitrate-free bacon

2 cups button mushrooms

1 medium onion (yellow or white)

2 celery stalks

2 carrots

2 cups pearl onions (peeled)

3 garlic cloves

2 tablespoons organic tomato paste

1/4 cup tapioca flour (arrowroot powder)

6 sprigs fresh thyme

1 bay leaf

1 teaspoon ground black pepper

2 teaspoons Celtic sea salt

2 tablespoons coconut oil (for cooking)

INSTRUCTIONS

1. Heat large skillet over medium-high heat. Add coconut oil to hot pan.

2. Chop or cube bacon and add to hot pan. Sauté until just crisp and fat renders out, about 5 - 8 minutes. Set aside in slow cooker.

3. Cut chicken into on-the-bone serving pieces (legs, wings, thighs, breasts). Then add to large mixing bowl. Season chicken with salt and pepper, then add tapioca or arrowroot. Toss to coat.

4. Shake off excess flour and add seasoned chicken to hot greased pan in batches to brown, about 4 minutes per side. Set aside in slow cooker.

5. Peel and quarter yellow or white onion. Peel and smash garlic. Quarter mushrooms. Add to hot pan and sauté about 5 minutes. Set aside in slow cooker.

6. Cut carrots and celery into quarters. Add to hot pan with peeled pearl onions, tomato paste, remaining tapioca or arrowroot, and chicken stock. Stir to combine and deglaze pan. Bring to simmer, about 5 minutes.

7. Pour mixture into slow cooker. Add red wine, bay leaf and fresh thyme. Stir to combine.

8. Cover slow cooker with lid. Turn on to low and cook 6 - 8 hours, until meat and veggies are tender.

9. Turn off slow cooker and carefully remove lid. Remove celery, carrot, thyme and bay leaf.

10. Transfer to serving dish and serve hot.

Uptown Clam Chowder

Prep Time: 10 minutes

Cook Time: 1 hour 15 minutes

Servings: 4

INGREDIENTS

24 - 36 medium live littleneck clams (or other clam varieties)

2 cans (11.5) organic tomato juice (or about 6 large tomatoes)

2 cans (14.5 oz) organic crushed tomatoes

2 medium carrots

2 medium celery stalks

2 medium parsnips

1 red bell pepper

1 tablespoon tamari (or coconut aminos or liquid aminos)

1 bay leaf

1/4 teaspoon cayenne pepper

1/2 teaspoon onion powder

1 tablespoon dried oregano

1 tablespoon dried basil

1 teaspoon dried thyme

1 teaspoon ground black pepper

Celtic sea salt, to taste

1 cup clam juice (or veggie or chicken stock, or water) (optional)

INSTRUCTIONS

1. Have fishmonger shuck clams. Or carefully shuck clams yourself. Reserve clam juice. Set aside in refrigerator.
2. Juice tomatoes, if using. Add tomato juice and crushed tomatoes to medium pot. Heat pot over high heat.
3. Remove seeds, stems and veins from bell pepper. Dice bell pepper, carrot, celery, and parsnips. Add to pot with spices and salt, to taste.
4. Bring pot to boil, then reduce heat to low. Place lid loosely over pot to prevent splatter. Simmer for 45 minutes. Stir occasionally.
5. Remove lid and stir. Add clam juice, stock or water to reach desired consistency (optional).
6. Remove clams from refrigerator and chop, if desired. Add clams and juice to pot. Stir to combine.
7. Replace lid and continue cooking about 20 - 30 minutes. Stir occasionally.
8. Transfer to serving dish and serve hot.

Holiday Baked Ham

Prep Time: 10 minutes

Cook Time: 5 hours

Servings: 12

INGREDIENTS

1 (12 lb) bone-in ham

1 (20 oz) can organic pineapple rings (in juice)

1/2 cup date butter (or raw honey or agave)

1/2 cup whole cloves

1/2 cup water

1 lemon

1 lime

1 orange

About 12 pitted cherries (optional)

Toothpicks (optional)

INSTRUCTIONS

1. Preheat oven to 325 degrees F.

2. Drain pineapple juice into small mixing bowl. Juice lemon, lime and orange into bowl. Add sweetener and water. Mix well.

3. Place ham in roasting pan and score rind in crosshatch (diamond) pattern with knife.

4. Press cloves into rind. Place cherries on rind and secure with toothpick. Hang pineapple rings on cherries.

5. Pour pineapple juice mixture over ham and bake uncovered 4 - 5 hours, until internal temperature reaches 160 degrees F. Baste with juices about every 30 minutes.

Remove ham from oven. Remove toothpicks and carve. Serve hot.

Snack Recipes

Crisp Sesame Crackers

Veggie Flax Crackers

Avocado Cashew Hummus with Cucumber

Sundried Tomato Cashew Hummus with Carrots

Cocoa Date Spread

Cashew Spinach Dip with Bell Pepper

Chocolate Hazelnut Spread with Apples

Cashew Butter Date Snacks

Very Cherry Energy Bars

Sweet Coconut Ambrosia Salad

Sweet Carrot Raisin Salad

Sweet Coconut Rice with Mango

Sweet Almond Crunch Cookies

Chewy Ginger Cookies

Chocolate Dusted Almonds

Chocolate Chia Pudding

Coconut Rice Pudding

Nori with Almond Cheese

Quick Asian Slaw

Awesome Strawberry Salsa

Supreme Mango Salsa

Hot Apricot Pineapple Salsa

Fresh Zesty Pico de Gallo

Holy Loaded Guacamole

Spicy Stuffed Jalapeños

Crisp Sesame Crackers

Prep Time: 10 minutes

Dehydrating Time: 12 - 20 hours

Servings: 4

INGREDIENTS

2 cups ground flax seed

2/3 cup whole flax seed

1 1/3 cups raw sunflower seeds

1/2 cup raw black sesame seeds (or white sesame seeds)

Small bunch fresh parsley

1/4 teaspoon dried basil

1/4 teaspoon onion powder

1/4 teaspoon garlic powder

1 teaspoon Celtic sea salt

2 2/3 cups water

INSTRUCTIONS

1. Place parchment paper or dehydrator sheets on two dehydrator trays.
2. Finely mince fresh parsley. Add to large mixing bowl with seeds, salt and spices. Mix until well combined.
3. Spread batter on prepared sheets. Place trays in dehydrator and set to 120 degrees F for 1 hour. Reduce temperature to 105 degrees F for remainder of dehydrating time.

4. After 4 hours dehydrating time, remove trays from dehydrator and use knife to score crackers in preferred shape and size. Place back in dehydrator and continue dehydrating another 4 hours.

5. Remove trays from dehydrator. Peel crackers from sheets and break apart along score lines. Place crackers directly on dehydrator tray and continue dehydrating another 4 - 12 hours, depending on desired crispness.

6. Remove crackers from dehydrator and serve with your favorite raw dips, spreads and salsas. Or store in an airtight container up to 4 weeks.

Veggie Flax Crackers

Prep Time: 10 minutes

Cook Time: 12 - 24 hours

Servings: 4

INGREDIENTS

1 medium tomato

1 medium onion

2 medium zucchini

1 cup ground flax seed

2 tablespoons coconut aminos (or raw apple cider vinegar)

1/2 teaspoon ground black pepper

1 teaspoon Celtic sea salt

INSTRUCTIONS

1. Place parchment paper or dehydrator sheets on two dehydrator trays.
2. Peel onion and chop. Chop zucchini and tomato. Add to food processor or high-speed blender with flax meal, coconut aminos or vinegar, salt and pepper. Process until well ground, about 2 minutes.
3. Spread batter on prepared sheets. Place trays in dehydrator and set to 120 degrees F for 1 hour. Reduce temperature to 105 degrees F for remainder of dehydrating time.
4. After 4 hours dehydrating time, remove trays from dehydrator and use knife to score crackers in preferred shape and size. Place back in dehydrator and continue dehydrating another 4 hours.

5. Remove trays from dehydrator. Peel crackers from sheets and break apart along score lines. Place crackers directly on dehydrator tray and continue dehydrating another 4 - 12 hours, depending on desired crispness.

6. Remove crackers from dehydrator and serve with your favorite raw dips, spreads and salsas. Or store in an airtight container up to 4 weeks.

Avocado Cashew Hummus with Cucumber

Prep Time: 5 minutes*

Servings: 4

INGREDIENTS

1 cup raw cashews

1 avocado

Juice of 1/2 lemon

2 garlic cloves

1 teaspoon ground white pepper (or 1/2 teaspoon ground black pepper)

Small bunch fresh cilantro

1/2 teaspoon Celtic sea salt

1 small cucumber

Water

INSTRUCTIONS

1. *Soak cashews in enough water to cover at least 4 hours, or overnight in refrigerator. Drain and rinse.
2. Peel garlic. Juice lemon. Remove cilantro leaves from stem. Add to food processor or high-speed blender with soaked cashews, salt and pepper.
3. Slice avocado in half. Remove pit and scoop flesh into processor. Process until smooth, about 1 - 2 minutes. Add water or raw oil to reach desired consistency, if necessary.
4. Transfer mixture to serving dish.

5. Peel cucumber if desired. Cut diagonally into 1/3 inch slices. Arrange on serving dish.

6. Serve immediately with hummus. Or place in refrigerator for 20 minutes, then serve chilled.

Sundried Tomato Cashew Hummus with Carrots

Prep Time: 5 minutes*

Servings: 4

INGREDIENTS

1 1/2 cup raw cashews

1/4 cup sundried tomatoes

1/4 cup raw tahini (or 1/3 cup raw sesame seeds)

1/2 lemon

1 small garlic clove

1 teaspoon ground white pepper (or 1/2 teaspoon ground black pepper)

1/2 teaspoon Celtic sea salt

2 large carrots

Water

INSTRUCTIONS

1. *Soak cashews in enough water to cover at least 4 hours, or overnight in refrigerator. Drain and rinse.
2. Peel garlic. Juice lemon. Add to food processor or high-speed blender with raw sesame seeds and process until smooth, if using.
3. Or add tahini to processor with soaked cashews, sundried tomatoes, garlic, lemon juice, salt and pepper. Process until smooth, about 1 - 2 minutes. Add water or raw oil to reach desired consistency, if necessary.
4. Transfer mixture to serving dish.

7. Peel carrots if desired. Cut into 4 inch long x 1/2 inch thick sticks. Arrange on serving dish.

5. Serve immediately with hummus. Or place in refrigerator for 20 minutes, then serve chilled.

Cocoa Date Spread

Prep Time: 5 minutes*

Servings: 4

INGREDIENTS

10 - 12 oz dried pitted dates

2 cups water

3 tablespoons raw cocoa powder

1/2 teaspoon ground cinnamon

1/4 teaspoon ground ginger

Ground black pepper, to taste

INSTRUCTIONS

1. *Soak dates in water overnight. Drain and reserve 1/4 cup liquid.

2. Add soaked dates, cocoa powder, cinnamon, ginger and black pepper to taste to food processor or high-speed blender. Pulse until chunky mixture forms. Add reserved liquid to reach desired consistency, if necessary.

3. Or add dates to medium mixing bowl with cocoa powder, cinnamon, ginger and black pepper to taste. Mash with large fork or potato masher for about 5 minutes, until chunky mixture forms. Add reserved liquid to reach desired consistency, if necessary.

4. Transfer to serving dish and serve with fruits, veggies, or raw crackers and breads.

Cashew Spinach Dip with Bell Pepper

Prep Time: 10 minutes

Servings: 2

INGREDIENTS

2 - 3 cups spinach leaves

1 1/2 cups raw cashews

3 garlic cloves

1 lemon

1/3 cup water

1/4 teaspoon mustard powder (or mustard seeds)

1/2 teaspoon ground white pepper (or 1/4 teaspoon ground black pepper)

1/2 teaspoon Celtic sea salt

1 red bell pepper

INSTRUCTIONS

1. Cut bell pepper in half and remove seeds, veins and stems. Slice peppers into 1 - 1 1/2 inch strips. Arrange on serving dish and set aside.

2. Juice lemon. Peel garlic. Add to food processor or high-speed blender with cashews and mustard powder or seeds. Process until finely ground, about 2 minutes.

3. Add salt, pepper and water. Process until smooth. Add spinach and pulse until spinach is desired texture.

4. Transfer mixture to serving dish. Serving immediately with bell pepper slices. Or refrigerate 20 minutes and serve chilled.

Chocolate Hazelnut Spread with Apples

Prep Time: 5 minutes*

Servings: 2

INGREDIENTS

1 cup raw hazelnuts

1/4 cup raw cocoa powder

1/4 cup raw honey (or dried pitted dates)

2/3 teaspoon vanilla

1/4 teaspoon Celtic sea salt

2 apples

Raw nut milk (optional)

Water

INSTRUCTIONS

8. *Soak hazelnuts in enough water to cover overnight in refrigerator. Soak dates in enough water to cover overnight in refrigerator, if using. Drain and rinse.

9. Add soaked hazelnuts to food processor or high-speed blender and process until smooth, up to 10 minutes. Scrape down sides as needed.

10. Add honey or soaked dates, cocoa powder, vanilla and salt. Process until smooth, about 1 minute. Add nut milk to reach desired consistency, if necessary.

11. Transfer mixture to serving dish.

12. Remove core, seeds and stems from apples. Slice into wedges and arrange on serving dish. Serve immediately.

Cashew Butter Date Snacks

Prep Time: 5 minutes

Servings: 2

INGREDIENTS

6 whole dried pitted dates

Pinch ground cinnamon

Raw Cashew Butter

1 cup raw cashews

1 dried pitted date

1 teaspoon raw oil (coconut, walnut, almond, sesame, etc.)

1/2 teaspoon ground cinnamon

1/4 teaspoon Celtic sea salt

(or 1/2 cup prepared raw cashew butter)

INSTRUCTIONS

1. For *Cashew Butter*, add cashews, date, cinnamon, salt and oil to food processor or high-speed blender. Process until smooth, up to 5 minutes. Let mixture rest between periods of processing to reach desired consistency, if necessary.

2. Slice dates in half lengthwise. Use small spoon to fill date halves with prepared or *Raw Cashew Butter*. Sprinkle ground cinnamon over filled dates.

3. Arrange on serving dish and serve immediately.

Very Cherry Energy Bars

Prep Time: 25 minutes

Servings: 6

INGREDIENTS

1 cup dried cherries

1/4 cup dried pitted dates

1 cup raw almonds

1/4 teaspoon ground cinnamon

1/4 teaspoon vanilla

1/8 teaspoon Celtic sea salt

1/3 cup warm water

1/2 sour orange (or orange or tangerine)

INSTRUCTIONS

1. Zest and juice orange into small mixing bowl. Add warm water and dried cherries. Toss to coat and set aside 10 minutes.

2. Line loaf pan with parchment paper.

3. Add nuts and dates to food processor or high-speed blender. Drain soaked cherries and add to processor with cinnamon, vanilla and salt. Process for about 1 minute, until mixture is coarsely ground and sticks together when pressed.

4. Scrape mixture into prepared loaf pan and press firmly into bottom with hands or spatula.

5. Place in refrigerator and chill for 10 minutes. Remove and cut into 6 bars.

6. Serve immediately. Or store in refrigerator up to 2 weeks.

Sweet Coconut Ambrosia Salad

Prep Time: 15 minutes*

Servings: 2

INGREDIENTS

3 mature coconuts

1 1/2 cups water

6 clementines or tangerines (about 1 cup segments)

1 cup fresh pineapple (chopped)

1 cup pecans (chopped)

1 cup fresh cherries (pitted)

INSTRUCTIONS

1. Remove coconut flesh from shells. Add 1 coconut and water to food processor or high-speed blender. Process until well blended and fairly smooth, about 1 - 2 minutes.

2. Strain mixture through nut milk bag, cheesecloth or strainer into container. Add coconut milk back to blender with flesh of 2nd coconut. Process again until well blended and thick, about 1 - 2 minutes.

3. Strain mixture through nut milk bag, cheesecloth or strainer into container. Reserve pulp and set aside to dry and dehydrate, then use as coconut flour.

4. *For thicker coconut cream, set aside thickened milk in refrigerator about 20 minutes and allow fat to separate. Remove coconut cream from refrigerator and scoop out risen fat into medium mixing bowl.

5. Or add coconut cream milk to medium mixing bowl. Peel oranges or tangerines and remove segments. Peel pineapple and chop. Cut cherries in half and pit. Chop pecans. Add to coconut cream.

6. Add remaining coconut flesh to clean food processor with shredding attachment and process, or grate with grater. Add coconut to mixture. Stir to combine.

7. Cover mixture and place in refrigerator for 2 hours. Remove and transfer to serving dishes.

8. Serve chilled.

Sweet Carrot Raisin Salad

Prep Time: 5 minutes

Servings: 2

INSTRUCTIONS

2 large carrots

2 tablespoons red raisins

2 tablespoons golden raisins

1/4 cup raw slivered almonds (or sliced almonds)

1/2 small orange (or tangerine)

1/4 teaspoon ground cinnamon

DIRECTIONS

1. Add carrots to food processor with shredding attachment and process, or grate with grater. Add to medium mixing bowl with raisins, almonds and cinnamon.
2. Zest *then* juice orange. Add to carrot mixture and toss to combine.
3. Transfer to serving dishes and serve immediately. Or refrigerate 20 minutes and serve chilled.

Sweet Coconut Rice with Mango

Prep Time: 10 minutes*

Servings: 2

INSTRUCTIONS

1 fresh coconut (or 2/3 cup desiccated, shredded or flaked coconut)

1/4 cup raw honey (or 1/4 cup dried pitted dates)

1/4 teaspoon ground ginger(or 1/4 inch piece fresh ginger)

1 mango

INGREDIENTS

1. *Soak dried coconut and dried pitted dates in enough water to cover overnight in refrigerator, if using. Drain coconut and add to medium mixing bowl. Drain dates and reserve 2 tablespoons soaking liquid.

2. Or remove fresh coconut flesh from shell and add to food processor with shredding attachment and process, or grate with grater. Add to medium mixing bowl.

3. Add soaked dates and soaking liquid to clean food processor or high-speed and process until smooth, if using.

4. Peel fresh ginger and mince or finely grate, if using. Add raw honey or date purée to shredded coconut with ground or fresh ginger. Mix to combine. Transfer to serving dishes.

5. Slice mango in half around pit. Remove peel and dice or thinly slice flesh. Add over sweet shredded coconut.

6. Serve immediately. Or refrigerate 20 minutes and serve chilled.

Sweet Almond Crunch Cookies

Prep Time: 20 minutes

Servings: 12

INGREDIENTS

3/4 cup raw almond butter (or 1 cup raw almonds)

2 - 4 tablespoons raw honey (or 1/4 cup dried pitted dates)

1 tablespoon ground chia seed or flax meal (or whole seeds)

1 teaspoon cinnamon

1/2 teaspoon Celtic sea salt

1/4 cup raw almonds

INSTRUCTIONS

11. Line baking dish with parchment paper.

12. Add 1/4 cup raw almonds to food processor or high-speed blender and process until finely chopped. Set aside.

13. Add whole chia or flax seeds to high-speed blender or spice grinder and grind to fine powder, if using.

14. Add chia or flax meal to food processor or high-speed blender with remaining almonds or almond butter, honey or dates, cinnamon and salt. Process until smooth, thick paste forms, up to 5 minutes. Let mixture rest between periods of processing to reach desired consistency, if necessary.

15. Spread mixture in parchment lined dish. Place in refrigerator or freezer for 10 minutes.

16. Remove dish and scoop with tablespoon or melon baller. Roll into balls with hands.

17. Place chopped almonds in shallow dish and roll balls in almonds to coat.

18. Transfer coated almond cookies to serving dish. Serve immediately. Or refrigerate 20 minutes and serve chilled.

Chewy Ginger Cookies

Prep Time: 20 minutes*

Servings: 12

INGREDIENTS

1/2 cup raw cashews (frozen)

1 1/2 cups dried pitted dates (1 cup chopped)

2 inch piece fresh ginger

1 teaspoon ground ginger

1/4 teaspoon ground cinnamon

1/2 cup unsweetened flaked or shredded coconut

INSTRUCTIONS

1. * Place cashews in freezer for a few hours to overnight.
2. Add frozen nuts to food processor or high-speed blender. Pulse until coarsely ground.
3. Peel and finely grate fresh ginger. Add to processor with dates, ground ginger and cinnamon. Process until mixture is well broken down and sticks together.
4. Form mixture into 12 balls. Add coconut flakes to shallow dish. Roll balla in coconut until well coated, then gently press to flatten slightly.
5. Arrange on serving dish and cover. Place in freezer for at least 10 minutes, until set up and firm.
6. Remove from freezer and serve chilled. Or store in freezer or refrigerator.

Chocolate Dusted Almonds

Prep Time: 20 minutes*

Servings: 2

INGREDIENTS

1 cup raw almonds

1 tablespoon raw cocoa powder

1 tablespoon raw honey

1/8 teaspoon ground cinnamon

1/8 teaspoon vanilla

INSTRUCTIONS

1. Add almonds and honey to small mixing bowl and toss to combine.
2. Add cocoa, cinnamon and vanilla and toss to evenly coat.
3. Transfer to serving dish and serve immediately.

Chocolate Chia Pudding

Prep Time: 15 minutes

Servings: 2

INGREDIENTS

1 cup nut milk (or 2 mature coconuts + 1 1/2 cups water)

2 - 4 tablespoons raw honey (or dried pitted dates)

2 - 4 tablespoons whole chia seeds

2 - 3 tablespoons cocoa powder

1/2 teaspoon vanilla

INSTRUCTIONS

1. Remove coconut flesh from shells. Add 1 coconut and water to food processor or high-speed blender. Process until well blended and fairly smooth, about 1- 2 minutes.

2. Strain mixture through nut milk bag, cheesecloth or strainer into container. Add coconut milk back to blender with remaining coconut flesh. Process again until well blended and fairly smooth, about 1 minute.

3. Strain mixture through nut milk bag, cheesecloth or strainer into container. Reserve pulp and set aside to dry and dehydrate, then use as coconut flour.

4. Add nut milk to high-speed blender with dates and process until smooth, if using.

5. Or add nut milk to small mixing bowl with honey or stevia, cocoa powder, vanilla and chia seeds. Whisk to combine. Set aside to thicken, about 1 minute.

6. Pour mixture into serving dishes and serve immediately. Or refrigerate 20 minutes and serve chilled.

Coconut Rice Pudding

Prep Time: 20 minutes

Servings: 4

INGREDIENTS

3 fresh coconuts (or 2 cups unsweetened flaked or shredded coconut)

1 cup water

1/4 - 1/2 cup raw honey (or dried pitted dates)

1 teaspoon vanilla

Water

INSTRUCTIONS

1. *Soak 1 1/2 cups flaked coconut and dates in enough water to cover in refrigerator overnight. Then drain, if using.
2. Or remove fresh coconut flesh from shells.
3. Add flesh of 1 fresh coconut or 3/4 cup soaked coconut, and water to high-speed blender. Process until well blended and fairly smooth, about 1- 2 minutes.
4. Strain mixture through nut milk bag, cheesecloth or strainer into container. Add coconut milk back to blender with flesh of 1 fresh coconut or remaining soaked coconut. Process again until well blended and fairly smooth, about 1 minute.
5. Strain mixture through nut milk bag, cheesecloth or strainer into container. Reserve pulp and set aside to dry and dehydrate, then use as coconut flour.
6. Add coconut cream, soaked dates and vanilla to food processor or high-speed blender. Process until smooth, about 1 minute.

7. Or add coconut cream to medium mixing bowl with raw honey and vanilla.

8. Add remaining fresh coconut flesh to food processer with shredding attachment and process, or shred with grater.

9. Add shredded fresh coconut or flaked coconut to coconut cream mixture and whisk until well combined.

10. Pour into serving dishes and serve immediately. Or refrigerate for 20 minutes and serve chilled.

Nori with Almond Cheese

Prep Time: 15 minutes*

Servings: 2

INGREDIENTS

4 - 6 sheets dried nori (seaweed paper)

Almond cheese

1 cup raw almonds

2 tablespoons raw oil (coconut, walnut, almond, sesame, etc.)

2 tablespoons lemon juice (or raw apple cider vinegar)

1 garlic clove

1/4 teaspoon paprika

1/4 teaspoon ground white pepper (or ground black pepper)

1/2 teaspoon Celtic sea salt

Water

INSTRUCTIONS

1. *For *Almond Cheese*, soak almonds in enough water to cover overnight. Drain and rinse. Pop off skins and discard.

2. Peel garlic and add to food processor or high-speed blender with soaked almonds, oil, lemon juice and/or vinegar, salt and spices. Process until smooth, about 2 minutes. Add water to reach desired consistency, if necessary.

3. Transfer mixture to small serving dish. Cut nori into small sheets and arrange on serving dish.

4. Serve immediately. Or refrigerate for 20 minutes and serve chilled.

Quick Asian Slaw

Prep Time: 15 minutes*

Servings: 4

INGREDIENTS

1/2 head red cabbage (2 cups shredded)

2 broccoli stalks (2 cups shredded)

1/4 cup dried cranberries

1/4 cup raw sliced or slivered almonds

2 tablespoons raw sunflower seeds

2 green onions (scallions)

1 carrot

1 lemon

1/2 orange

2 tablespoons raw honey

2 tablespoons raw sesame oil (or coconut, walnut, almond oil, etc.)

2 tablespoons apple cider vinegar

1/2 teaspoon ground ginger

1 teaspoon ground white pepper (or black pepper)

1 teaspoon Celtic sea salt

INSTRUCTIONS

1. Add broccoli and carrot to food processor with shredding attachment, or grate with grater. Slice green onions. Shred cabbage. Add to large mixing bowl.

2. Add cranberries, almonds, sunflower seeds, honey, oil, vinegar, ginger, salt, pepper and squeeze of lemon and orange. Mix until well combined.

3. *Transfer mixture and for 90 minutes. Serve chilled.

Awesome Strawberry Salsa

Prep Time: 5 minutes*

Servings: 4

INGREDIENTS

2 cups fresh strawberries

1/2 small white onion

1/4 red bell pepper

Medium bunch fresh mint

1/2 lime

1/2 orange

1/2 teaspoon ground black pepper

INSTRUCTIONS

1. Remove strawberry stems and leaves, then finely dice. Add to medium mixing bowl.

2. Peel onion and finely dice. Remove mint leave s from stem then chiffon, or thinly slice. Add to strawberries with pepper and squeeze of lime and orange. Mix until well combined.

3. Transfer mixture to serving dish and serve immediately with raw chips. Or refrigerate for 20 minutes and serve chilled.

Supreme Mango Salsa

Prep Time: 10 minutes

Servings: 4

INGREDIENTS

2 mangos

1/4 small red onion

1/4 red bell pepper

Small bunch fresh cilantro

1 lime

1/2 fresh jalapeño pepper

1/4 teaspoon Celtic sea salt

INSTRUCTIONS

1. Slice mangos in half around pit. Remove peel and finely dice flesh. Add to medium mixing bowl.

2. Peel onion and dice. Remove seeds, stem and vein from bell pepper, then finely dice. Finely chop cilantro. Remove seeds and stem from jalapeño, then mince. Add to mango with salt and squeeze of lime. Mix until well combined

3. Transfer mixture to serving dish and serve immediately with raw chips. Or refrigerate for 20 minutes and serve chilled.

Hot Apricot Pineapple Salsa

Prep Time: 15 minutes

Servings: 4

INGREDIENTS

1 cup fresh pineapple (diced)

3 fresh apricots

1/2 green bell pepper

1/2 cup cherry tomatoes

2 shallots

2 garlic cloves

1 lime

1 fresh Serrano pepper

Small bunch cilantro leaves

1/2 teaspoon cayenne pepper

1/4 teaspoon Celtic sea salt

INSTRUCTIONS

1. Peel pineapple and finely dice. Cut apricots in half and remove pits, then finely dice. Add to medium mixing bowl.

2. Peel shallots and thinly slice. Peel garlic and mince or thinly slice. Remove seeds, stem and vein from bell pepper, then finely dice. Quarter cherry tomatoes. Add to pineapple and apricot.

3. Finely chop cilantro. Remove seeds and stem from Serrano pepper, then mince. Add to bowl with salt, cayenne and squeeze of lime. Mix until well combined.

4. Transfer mixture to serving dish and serve immediately with raw chips. Or refrigerate for 20 minutes and serve chilled.

Fresh Zesty Pico de Gallo

Prep Time: 15 minutes*

Servings: 4

INGREDIENTS

4 plum tomatoes

1/2 small red onion

Small bunch fresh cilantro

1/2 jalapeño pepper

1/2 lime

1 garlic clove

1/8 teaspoon garlic powder

1/4 teaspoon ground cumin

1/4 teaspoon Celtic sea salt

1/4 teaspoon ground black pepper

INSTRUCTIONS

1. Finely dice tomatoes. Peel and dice onion. Add to medium mixing bowl.
2. Finely chop cilantro. Remove seeds, veins and stem from jalapeño, then mince. Peel and mince garlic. Add to tomatoes with salt, spices and squeeze of lime. Mix until well combined.
3. Transfer mixture to serving dish
4. *Refrigerate 3 hours. Serve room temperature or chilled with raw chips.

Holy Loaded Guacamole

Prep Time: 5 minutes

Servings: 2

INGREDIENTS

2 ripe avocados

1 small plum tomato

1/4 small red onion

Medium bunch fresh cilantro

1/2 lime

1/2 teaspoon smoked paprika

1/2 teaspoon ground black pepper

1/2 teaspoon Celtic sea salt

INSTRUCTIONS

1. Cut avocados in half and remove pits. Scoop flesh into small mixing bowl.
2. Peel onion and dice. Dice tomato. Finely chop cilantro. Add to avocado with salt, spices, and squeeze of lime. Mash with fork until well combined.
3. Transfer mixture to serving dish and serve immediately with raw chips. Or refrigerate for 20 minutes and serve chilled.

Spicy Stuffed Jalapeños

Prep Time: 15 minutes*

Dehydrating Time: 8 - 24 hours

Servings: 4

INGREDIENTS

6 fresh jalapeño peppers

1 cup raw sunflower seeds

1/2 cup water

1/4 cup nutritional yeast

1 lemon

2 teaspoons onion powder

1/2 teaspoon cayenne pepper

1 teaspoon Celtic sea salt

Water

INSTRUCTIONS

1. *Soak sunflower seeds in enough water to cover for 2 hours. Drain and rinse.

2. Cut jalapeños in half lengthwise and remove stems, seeds and veins. Place peppers on dehydrator tray.

3. Juice lemon. Add to food processor or high-speed blender with soaked sunflower seeds, water, nutritional yeast, salt, pepper and spices. Process until thick, smooth paste forms, about 2 minutes.

4. Fill piping bag with mixture and pipe into jalapeño halves. Or use teaspoon to scoop filling into jalapeño halves.

5. Place stuffed peppers on dehydrator sheets filling-side up. Set dehydrator to 110 degrees F for 8 - 24 hours, depending on desired texture.

6. Remove peppers from dehydrator and serve immediately.